Jeremy Whittle

BAD BLOOD

The Secret Life of the Tour de France

YELLOW JERSEY PRESS
LONDON

Published by Yellow Jersey Press 2009

6 8 10 9 7

Copyright © Jeremy Whittle 2008

Jeremy Whittle has asserted his right under the Copyright,
Designs and Patents Act 1988 to be identified as the author of this work

First published in Great Britain in 2008 by
Yellow Jersey Press
Random House, 20 Vauxhall Bridge Road,
London SW1V 2SA

www.rbooks.co.uk

Addresses for companies within The Random House Group Limited can be found at:
www.randomhouse.co.uk/offices.htm

The Random House Group Limited Reg. No. 954009

A CIP catalogue record for this book
is available from the British Library

ISBN 9780224080231

The Random House Group Limited supports The Forest Stewardship Council®
(FSC®), the leading international forest certification organisation. All our titles that are
printed on Greenpeace approved FSC® certified paper carry the FSC® logo. Our paper
procurement policy can be found at www.randomhouse.co.uk/environment

Typeset in Bembo by Palimpsest Book Production Ltd
Grangemouth, Stirlingshire
Printed in the UK by CPI Bookmarque, Croydon, CR0 4TD

For D and E

BAD BLOOD

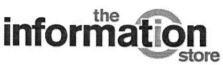
Tribune. He has appeared on BBC, NPR and CNN and is the author of *Yellow Fever* (1998) and *Le Tour* (2003). *Bad Blood* was shortlisted for the William Hill Sports Book of the Year 2008.

Also by Jeremy Whittle

Yellow Fever
Le Tour

THE TRIAL OF MILLAR AND GAUMONT

On 6 November, 4, British cyclist David Millar went on trial in the Parisian suburb of Nanterre for doping offences.

Initially, Millar faced a heavy fine and the remote possibility of imprisonment. Not for the first time, Millar, who had already confessed to doping, was contrite and plain-speaking. The prosecution was sympathetic and dropped a demand for a custodial sentence.

Across the room, his estranged former Cofidis teammate, Philippe Gaumont, also facing charges, looked on. Gaumont, once an elite athlete, now ran a bar in Amiens and smoked heavily.

In January 2004, after he had first been interviewed by the French investigating judge, Richard Pallain, Gaumont returned home to his wife and two children. The Frenchman knew that what he had told Judge Pallain about rampant doping practices within cycling had made him unemployable. He had broken the omerta, the law of silence over doping that reigned within the sport. He was finished, cast out, his career as a cyclist over.

All day, as his arrest and its repercussions gathered pace, Gaumont's face had featured in TV news bulletins across France.

As he closed the front door behind him, exhausted by his ordeal, his five-year-old son ran excitedly into the hallway.

'I saw you on telly, Daddy!' he said. 'Did you win again? Can I see your medal?'

In the cupboard under the stairs in my house, I have a shelf crammed with frayed old maps. Most of them are of Europe, although there are some of the Lake District, the Brecon Beacons, the north Cornish coast and the South Downs.

One of them is a tattered French map, Michelin 245 (Provence-Côte d'Azur). It is torn from being stuffed hurriedly into the glovebox of hire cars, or into the back pocket of a sweat-soaked cycling jersey. It has been wrinkled by summer storms on hot evenings, frayed and ripped by the Mistral wind sweeping across the hills of the Vaucluse and stained by coffee spilt at unsteady pavement tables.

The many roads, criss-crossing vineyards and olive groves, tracing mountain passes and high gorges, are marked in red, yellow and white. They have become as familiar to me as the lines around my eyes. My Michelin 245 is now so well worn that it is falling apart, but it has particular sentimental value. This is not just because favourite routes, driven and ridden but now known by heart, are picked out in highlighter pen, but also because in the bottom corner, written in a precise and delicate hand, are directions to a discreet address in the smarter suburbs of Nice.

For a foreigner, with − certainly, back then − little grasp of the culture of his adopted home, Lance Armstrong's spelling of French names was precise:

Take the Grand Corniche, after 600m there is a road called Boulevard des Deux Corniches also there is a sign for a

school called Institut de Blanche de Castille, then go to
Ave Dillies.

Armstrong scribbled his address on my map in March 1999,
three months before he won his first Tour de France. We were
about to make a short film together to promote the Lance
Armstrong cancer foundation, and the second issue of *procycling*
magazine. He wrote the note as he sat in a hotel lobby in
Sisteron, describing the renovations to his new home while
cursing standards of French workmanship. We planned to film
a couple of days later at his villa, perched on a wooded hillside
overlooking Nice's jumble of red roofs. The house had spectacular views over the Côte d'Azur. In the distance, beyond the
promenade des Anglais, planes took off from Nice's international
airport, spinning out across the Mediterranean before they turned
north towards the Alps. From the terrace, there were panoramic
views towards a chain of morning-blue mountains rising up
from the coastline.

After six years' collaboration on magazine stories, newspaper
articles and ghosted columns, this was to be our final meaningful alliance. Within a year, his spiralling stardom and our differing
stances on cycling's war on doping had irreparably tainted our
relationship. Estranged from the French, his villa was soon sold
and he had moved on, to Girona in Spain.

This is the story of how the schism over doping ended not
only that friendship, but many others, as scandal after scandal
robbed European cycling of its credibility. As the polarisation
over doping took root, several of Armstrong's teammates, rivals
and associates were casualties of this war.

Between 1999 and 2005, cycling entered a period of unprecedented wealth as Armstrong himself constructed a parallel
universe of power and affluence. Yet the Armstrong era was book-
ended by the two great doping scandals of modern cycling: the
Festina Affair of 1998 and the Kafkaesque confusion of the unre-
solved Operacíon Puerto investigation in 2006. The Texan was

the iconic figure of these boom years, both as a cancer survivor and also as a survivor in a bitter ethical war that claimed careers and even lives.

The casualties of that conflict, lone voices who stood up against a culture of cheating, were driven underground, bullied out of their jobs and out of their sport. This is a story of those collapsed friendships, of back-stabbing and double-dealing, of polarised positions in the fight to purge sport of its ethical malaise. Finally, this is about my own journey from wide-eyed and unquestioning acceptance to dejected scepticism, as I witnessed opportunism, greed and bumbling bureaucracy reinforce the casual deceit of a generation of athletes and crush the hopes for redemption of a sport crippled by moral decay.

At first, following Europe's cycling circuit is a thrilling ride, a glamorous, multilingual, gypsy-like existence, a blur of airports and hotels, taxis and check-in desks; a road movie shot under blue skies in stunning locations, in pursuit of lean, tanned and beautiful athletes.

There is the seduction of each setting: Tuscany, Provence, Andalusia, California; the breakneck visits to Geneva, Bordeaux, Naples, Cordoba, San Francisco; the thrill of closed roads and cheering crowds; the snatched intimacies with those on the outside, who look, longingly, into the bubble, while cursing the tedium of their daily routines.

Yet, the European cycling circuit is so all-consuming that, even as a journalist, it can make a prisoner of you. In my case, it gave me a feeling of belonging, something that was missing from my life at the time. The real world slipped away; slowly but surely, I was seduced and became immersed in the sport. All that mattered to me was The Race. There are so many races, and some of them are so long – over three weeks for each of the 'grand tours' of France, Italy and Spain – that they develop a world of their own. When they end, you feel wrung out, battle weary, divorced from reality.

Even less important stage races such as Paris–Nice, Tirreno-Adriatico, the Tour de l'Avenir, usually last at least a week. Many journalists live and travel in this bubble with the teams and their personnel. Slowly but surely, the lines become blurred.

Journalists develop an intimacy with the riders that is rare in other sports. They catch the same flights as they shuttle from race to race; they stay in the same hotels; they bump into them in lifts or at breakfast buffets, exchanging greetings and a word or two of encouragement. They share their successes and failures, wince at their injuries, develop friendships with their families and – in one case I know of – transport their drugs for them.

Many of them suspect and often know far more than they reveal. Soon the *omerta*, the law of silence, governs their existence, just like it governs that of the riders. It is a closed, self-serving culture, a secret society, with its own unspoken rules. These rules are not those of the outside world.

It took a while for me to realise that doping was all-pervasive. For a long time the only evidence was anecdotal – a story of a coat borrowed from a team manager with a discarded syringe in the inside pocket, the nods and knowing smiles at an exceptional performance.

But then, all of the gypsies in the caravan are eking out a living from the sport, as riders, team personnel or media. Some are wealthy, but many are surviving, simply pleased to be there, cushioned from reality. On the road, everyday obligation – families and children, mortgages and bills, ethics and morality – slowly recedes.

That isolation is one of the motors of the strange siege mentality that surrounds cycling – the continuing attitude that the sport is almost beyond reproach, whatever happens, because unless you too have suffered through the Tour and the Giro, through Flanders and Roubaix, you 'wouldn't understand'.

For those whose long absences have caused cracks to appear in their domestic relationships, the sense of escape is what is most appealing. Cycling can be a solitary pursuit, embraced by those who dream of escape and freedom. Some of that sense of longing and loneliness is manifest in the hotel corridors and at the dining tables, where ex-pros, reluctant to let go, prolong the dream long after their own athletic careers have ended, hanging on as if they can't bear to leave. Cycling's escapist appeal is never better expressed than in the mountains and perhaps that is why they remain the most evocative terrain. The long climbs to each summit encapsulate the struggle to shake off the humdrum shackles of responsibility; the swooping frenetic descents into the valleys, the crazed exultation of freedom and escape.

Despite its romance, European cycling has never been able to penetrate the mainstream consciousness in the English-speaking world consistently. Interest flickers on and off, peaking in July when the Tour de France holds centre stage. Of contemporary stars, only Armstrong has become a household name and, stateside at least, that has been as much for his iconic and patriotic persona in the post-9/11 climate, as for his achievements on a bike.

Because of doping, my dream job, a job that gave me such a sense of escape, gradually imprisoned me. For a long time I refused to choose sides: it was easier, far easier, not to. Like others, I wanted to write about the glory and heroism of sport, but instead I became lost in the moral maze, an accomplice to the *omerta*, an accessory to the Big Lie.

Then, standing with my notebook and tape recorder, when a drugs ampoule fell at my feet, as a rider exhaustedly pulled his racing jersey over his head, my journey from fan to accomplice became complete.

'You weren't supposed to see that, Jeremy,' he smiled weakly. I stared at the floor. I didn't know what to say.

Eventually, I lifted my head and said: 'Don't worry.'

Even now, it is easier not to name that rider, partly because he is not a thoroughbred but an also-ran who has never won

6

a major race; partly because he is a 'good' guy with young children, who don't deserve to have their father labelled a cheat or to have abuse heaped on them when they arrive at school; and partly because I am still surprised at my own naivety in thinking that, for some reason, he was too nice a guy, *too good*, to be a doper.

One thing I have learned is this: nice, well educated and intelligent athletes, athletes with children and families, dogs and cats, athletes who give to charity and kiss babies, they lie and cheat too.

And then, I doped myself once, not for money, not for the pursuit of excellence or the purposes of research, but just to get to the finish. I was competing as a weekend warrior in the Paris-Roubaix cyclotourist event. This is not even a race, but a timed 'challenge', a test of endurance over 165 miles in northern France.

I'm not sure why that Paris-Roubaix felt so much worse than other similar events I'd ridden, up and down France, but it was. I remember the endless flat roads rolling north-east from Compiegne towards the Belgian border, the battle to pedal against a headwind over the cobblestone tracks crossing back and forth through the monochrome landscape, increasingly sharp stabs of tendinitis, a pulsating headache and then, finally, the desire to lie down on the pavement, thirty kilometres from the finish line in Roubaix's old and shabby velodrome.

'What's the matter?' the others asked, when we stopped at the final checkpoint.

'I'm wasted,' I whined, as I sat, head in hands, on the doorstep of a battered red-brick house somewhere on the Franco-Belgian border.

'Here.' An opened palm containing two small pills appeared in front of me. Without a second thought, without recourse to the ethical parameters of fair play that had been drilled into me by my middle-class parents and middle-class teachers at my middle-class school, I greedily popped the pills into my mouth. I can, in the style of Richard Virenque in a French courtroom, plead innocence and say I didn't know what I was taking, but that would be disingenuous. It would also be a lie.

Maybe it was the overall cheapness of the trip that caused my moral compass to spin out of control. But I can't really blame the snoring and farting in our pre-race dormitory accommodation for my fatigue, nor my sacrilegious choice of the Italian national champion's jersey for race day, which led to some multilingual and demoralising sledging from those who overtook me. Maybe like Laurent Fignon, whose pony-tail once cost him the Tour de France, it was my Michael Hutchence mane, a tumble of tresses that no Adidas headband could contain, that created too much drag and proved my undoing.

Whatever, the amphetamines did the trick.

Five minutes later, the world was in technicolour again. I sped down the road at the head of our small group. I felt no pain. I was reborn. I was a tiger. I was ecstatic, joyful, like a child running out of class at the end of the school day.

The fireworks didn't last long.

An hour or so later I pedalled, a spent force, into the Roubaix twilight, onto the banking of the old velodrome and, finally, across the finish line. As I slumped over the handlebars, I was mocked by another of our party, a pockmarked Yorkshirewoman with the physique of an Eastern Bloc shot-putter. That night I lay in bed, staring at the ceiling, wide-eyed and dehydrated, waiting for dawn. I was a red-eyed zombie on the coach back home.

Because of its institutionalised reliance on performance enhance-ment, European road racing has been at the cutting edge of the doping experience; no other sport has made accomplices of so many of its followers. Football, tennis, even athletics should think themselves lucky not to have been so publicly humiliated by an environment in which dope cheats have for so long been accepted and, in fact, allowed to flourish.

This acceptance of doping can be attributed to the long-established brutality of professional cycling, the endless pursuit of success, the pressure from rivals, the dangers of racing, the anonymity of anybody other than The Champion. By its nature, it is a sport filled with losers and also-rans, controlled by a minority of winners, who are paranoid about protecting their own status, terrified of humiliation and haunted by that sudden inexplicable loss of power that spells The End.

Ironically, it is that brutality and cruelty that makes it so seductive. It was that tradition of sacrifice and pain that reeled me in when in July 1985 I sat entranced, watching Channel 4's coverage of Bernard Hinault's final Tour victory. As a sports fan, that year's Tour was an epiphany. But in the two decades since then, and particularly in the aftermath of Greg LeMond's three Tour wins, there was a unique opportunity for a more sinister culture of doping to develop. During my time reporting on the sport, cycling has demonstrated the ethics of a banana republic, with corruption and despotic behaviour on an unprecedented level. The technological extent of that chicanery has been painstakingly documented elsewhere.

I am not a scientist or an authority on the technicalities of doping. I do not set out to prove that cycling has a chronic doping problem – the sport itself has ably demonstrated that. But I believe that sport has as much of a role to play in the fabric of our lives as politics or art, and what interests me is not a litany of naming and shaming but the effect of a tacit acceptance of institutionalised doping, both on professional athletes and on their fans. What does living this lie do to athletes and their families? How do they cope with the real world once their fraudulent careers are over? How do you rediscover your love of sport when it has been betrayed by doping?

I was – and remain – a sports fan who, through a happy accident, became a sports journalist. In the past, I have been as moved by the Tour de France as by anything in my life. The unpalatable truth, for me and for anyone else who loves cycling, is that the event has now become synonymous with cheating.

9

So it is ironic that some within cycling may ostracise me because of this book. I was once a devoted pilgrim. I have read their stories and studied their videos and been moved by their suffering. I have ridden up mountain passes and stood at the roadsides for hours on end, frozen and hungry, just to cheer them on their way. They created an elemental part of me; they nurtured my obsession and fed my love of the sport. They were my heroes.

And it is so very hard to accept, so very hard indeed, when you learn that your heroes have feet of clay.

Part One

The Bike in the Hall

'There are three sides to every story: yours ... mine ...
and the truth.'

Robert Evans, *The Kid Stays In The Picture*

London, 1993

'Turn him around so he can see the sunset,' said Tom Dobson. Immediately behind the smirking shadow cabinet minister's son, Red Menace centre half David Milliband jogged over, cupped a hand to his mouth in horror and turned away.

I lay on my back on an AstroTurf football pitch in Battersea Park, my left leg crumpled beneath me. In the dusk, my teammates gathered and stood over me. I watched the clouds drift past. Birds sang in nearby trees. Our field of dreams grew dark as we waited for the ambulance.

The floodlights hummed and flickered on. A game of hockey on the adjacent pitch was momentarily halted as the blue flashing lights appeared. The players stared bemused across the pitch at the crumpled figure. 'Shiiit, that hurts,' I hissed as I gave up the struggle to get back on my feet. Paramedics lifted me gingerly onto the stretcher.

I had been on the pitch only a couple of minutes, taking up my usual midfield position just in front of 'Big Dave' Milliband. He will forgive me if I say he is a better potential prime minister than a centre half.

Milliband's calling card was his sheer size. He'd bellow a booming 'Dave's ball!' at every goal kick, regardless of his positioning. His forehead was a battering ram, sending each hopeful punt soaring back towards the opposition. We were captained by Dan Corry, a skipper blessed with the decisive leadership style of John Le Mesurier in *Dad's Army*, latterly best known for a fateful email exchange on 11 September, 2001.

The other positions in the team were filled by thrusting young Labourites. A hardened Sunday Leaguer and fully paid-up mockney, I swore more than the others – and certainly a lot more than Milliband. I was a ringer, with trademark mane and headband, brought in chiefly because I had some training bibs, spare shin pads – and took corners.

That spring evening, fate intervened. A ball lofted high over my head had bounced between us all. I pivoted, volleyed the ball away and, as I landed, heard the snap of my kneecap.

New Labour's ministerial hopefuls watched the ambulance leave. Unlike their glorious leader, there was to be no golden goodbye, no testimonial moment. My career in park football was finished. 'I think it's only dislocated,' I said to the nurse, as they drove me to the Accident and Emergency wing of St Stephen's Hospital in Fulham. 'Maybe you can put it back . . .?'

As we trundled over speed bumps in the south London back-streets, she did as I asked. Detached from the pain, a gas mask clamped to my face, I watched curiously as she manipulated my knee. It felt as if she was sifting shingle through her fingers.

Later, after more gas, the Sister scissored through my boots and socks. I reached for the gas mask again and grinned deliriously as they did it. They smeared a cast from my heel to my groin and wheeled me into a ward. As a weekend warrior, I was finished.

'Don't expect to play sport again,' the surgeon told me after the operation.

Not even cycling, I asked?

Maybe cycling, he said. Maybe – but not for a long time.

This, it has to be said, was a bit of a blow. I had no job and no prospects. Now I had no escape either. Sport had rescued me from isolation as a teenager and from jobless depression as an adult. As I was wheeled back to the ward through a vague fog of anaesthesia, the black dogs barked and howled.

The ever-cheery Tom Dobson came to my hospital room to watch the Cup Final. He smuggled in some cans of Stella in a carrier bag and gurned in mock revulsion when I showed him the scar. 'It was my ball anyway, Jezzer,' he said.

I wailed like a baby during the first agonising days of physiotherapy. Crutches, however, had their advantages. People held doors open and black-cab drivers, showing a rare glimmer of humanity, no longer refused the fare home, south of the river.

My crutches also became a prop. At a wedding in Edinburgh, the bride's mother looked appalled, as, drunk as a skunk, I played a crutch-wielding Kenny Rogers, hobbling through a karaoke version of 'Ruby, Don't Take Your Love To Town', relishing the line 'It's hard to love a man whose legs are bent and paralysed . . .' After a while, they gave me a walking stick. Between sessions of physio, I camped on the sofa and became an expert on daytime TV. Left leg perched on a chair, remote control at my side, I started writing. I wrote for magazines, any magazine, on everything from Vanessa Feltz and her monumental cleavage to Siberian oil and gas supplies. A trickle of cheques dropped through the letter box.

More than anything, I wanted to write about sport. The editor of a cycling magazine, a friend of a friend, gave me a break. Could I go to Yorkshire to interview a young American professional? I caught a train to Leeds, and anxiously limped down a hotel corridor, preparing to knock on Lance Armstrong's bedroom door.

Armstrong was a hothead from Texas who was threatening to take bike racing by storm. They said he had an attitude problem. They also said he was the future of the sport.

For a long time in my life, there were few things as inspiring as the Tour de France. I cherished the race and its long history. I measured the passing of time, not by Christmas and New Year, but by the annual excitement of the Tour. The grandeur and spectacle of the race, the names of the towns and the mountain passes, got under my skin as much as the sight of the sweat-streaked, glassy-eyed riders toiling across expansive ancient landscapes. I loved the fact that the Tour crossed mountain ranges, wide estuaries and endless plains, that the peloton flashed past road signs to Bordeaux and Geneva, Barcelona and Milan, Nice and Brussels. Now, they are all just over an hour from Stansted, Heathrow or Gatwick; yet twenty years ago, before cheap flights shrunk our world, the names still evoked a dizzying pan-European exoticism.

The Tour's tradition of *camaraderie et amité*, nobility and honour achieved through suffering and sacrifice, its against-all-the-odds nature, has an enduring appeal. Falling in love with the Tour led to falling in love with France.

Yet as I fell in love with their landmark sporting event, the French were growing restless. They were familiar, perhaps overly familiar, with the Tour's tall stories. They had become complacent and disenchanted, and they needed a steady flow of French champions to keep the dream alive.

In the mid 1980s the successes of a stream of English-speaking riders brought huge television audiences to the event, as a new world discovered the Tour's old myths and legends. Meanwhile, even as they embraced the influx of tourism and revenue from the Tour's bewitched new fans, the French took solace in their former glories. Year by year, as the foreign legion swamped their territory, their love of cycling faded.

By the turn of the decade, the battle lines were drawn between the old world and the new, between tradition and modernisation. The success of a young American called Greg LeMond had stirred interest on the other side of the Atlantic. LeMond had challenged Breton farmer's son Bernard Hinault, the last bastion of French tradition and, coincidentally, LeMond's mentor, in an epic 1986 Tour. LeMond stood the test to become the first American winner. The Tour was never the same again and Hinault, winner in 1985, remains the last French champion.

LeMond's sheer *Americanness* appalled French purists. He was an innovator who saw cycling as an old-fashioned business with potential for growth. He expected to be a high earner, he wanted his wife to travel with him, he ate ice cream and he demanded air conditioning in his hotel room. The outrage at his behaviour reached its peak when he once decided to play golf on the Tour's rest day. Pétanque, he might have got away with, but golf . . .? This was sacrilegious. What made him all the more remarkable was that LeMond was sponsored by a French team – led by Hinault – yet he still had the guts to break the mould. LeMond was a fan but also a foreigner, an outsider, *un étranger*, competing on his own terms, yet sensitive to European sensibilities. He learned to speak French and rode in Classic races such as Paris-Roubaix, in an effort to prove he was no dilettante. Nevertheless, his victory over Hinault, by then an iconic figure in French cultural life, broke the years of French resistance and ushered in a new era; incredibly, no native rider has won the Tour since. That's twenty-two years – and counting.

The American, still riding for European sponsors, went on to win the Tour twice more. Those who have followed in his wake, led by Armstrong, have been corporate athletes, mostly riding for American brands in American teams, with little time for cycling's history. They have surfed a wave of opportunity and created vast wealth for themselves and an entourage of hangers-on.

Armstrong was always keen to carve his own place in the sport and often sought to distance himself from LeMond's legacy. 'I'm not the next Greg LeMond – I'm the first Lance Armstrong,' he would say, a little impatiently, when he first made his mark in Europe.

Ignoring Floyd Landis and his 2006 'victory', quickly discredited by his positive drugs test, there have now been ten American wins, shared between LeMond and Armstrong, in the past twenty years. But it was Armstrong, the recovered cancer sufferer and tough-talking charity spokesman with his Hollywood friends and celebrity lovers, who became the poster boy for cycling's new world.

As Armstrong took the Tour by storm, winning for seven successive years, the French became sullen and resentful, taking refuge in the notion of two-speed cycling – one group of riders (principally themselves), was clean and credible; the other group, they preferred to think of as dirty and doped. They even coined a phrase for it, *cyclisme à deux vitesses*.

Meanwhile, they remain as distant from Tour success as ever.

HERRING FOR BREAKFAST

I knew virtually nothing of professional cycling until 1985 when I shared a flat with Peter The Architect.

Peter had a mountainous stash of bike mags – bike porn, his girlfriend called it – and an encyclopaedic knowledge of Campagnolo rear derailleurs. He knew the nicknames of all the top riders: Campionissimo, Blaireau, and less exotically, the Pocket Rocket and the Staffordshire Engine. He spent most of his time swanning around in cycling kit, usually black with a Campagnolo logo. For comfort reasons, but also perhaps for that certain frisson of anticipation, he often went 'commando', *sans* underwear. He argued that this made him more aerodynamic. He was a posh Jewish architecture student with no pants – on a bike.

Architects loved racing bikes. The post-Kraftwerk generation, all black shirts and geometric haircuts, loved cycling. They drooled over the simple purity, the clean construction – the minimalist efficiency of the machines. The clothing, defined by form and function, devoid of frippery and frills and created in cutting edge postmodernist materials, also met with their approval.

They would stand around leering at fancy lugwork and stroking the Velcro fastening on racing shoes, perving over bottom brackets and quick-release mechanisms. In fact, the biggest 'bike perv' of all among the goatee-sporting, Channel-4-watching, latte-slurping, risotto-eating design intelligentsia of the late 1980s, turned out to be Paul Smith, the charming English dandy from Nottingham, now a legend in menswear, who once aspired to be a professional racing cyclist.

While mountain bikes were common as muck, racing bikes were sexy, elitist, foreign. Owning one said a lot about you: you had almost certainly been abroad, you watched the Tour on Channel 4, maybe you spoke a little French, had a smattering of Italian, got your suits tailor-made in Soho, and you certainly knew where Bar Italia was. By the time we had all seen slow-motion footage of Bernard Hinault, sexy, dashing and Breton, swooping through the Alps in his Ray-Bans to the hypnotic beats of Kraftwerk's anthem, 'Tour de France' – which even got namechecked by Afrika Bambaataa and the Sugarhill Gang – cycling was officially cool, very cool indeed.

Peter and I became close friends when we shared a flat in Clapham. Bikes cluttered the hall. We ate curry and drank beer. We fitted the bike-loving architecture student stereotype. He worshipped Judge Dredd, while I loved Gil Scott-Heron. We admired Le Corbusier, Frank Gehry and Rem Koolhaas – not past winners of Paris-Roubaix or the Tour of Flanders, but groundbreaking design heroes. We wore a lot of black. We loved retro styling. In July, we fed our cycling obsession by watching the Tour on 4. At weekends we cleaned our bikes. Sometimes we even rode them. Peter's sparkling Roberts racing frame lived in his bedroom, leaning against the wall below the life-size posters of Francesco Moser and of course, Bernard Hinault.

We aspired to the physique of a Moser or Hinault, but knew little of their dietary regime. So we invented our own. Occasionally Peter began the day with a rollmop herring washed down with a can of Stella. I'd roll my eyes in mock disgust, while spreading marmalade on a bacon and Stilton sandwich.

Peter relentlessly fuelled my growing interest in cycling. He persuaded me to spend forty quid on a bike from a junk shop on Holloway Road. We rented *Breaking Away*, the cult American cycling movie, and slumped on the sofa, watching it again and again, until we could recite the script. I pottered around town on the bike, commuting from Clapham to Islington and back, gradually getting fitter and faster. I'd ride into the West End, cruise through Mayfair and Soho, climb up to Highgate and then head back home through Chelsea and Battersea, racing buses and taxis on the way.

Andy joined us on rides around Richmond Park. He was cooler than both of us because he had an aluminium-framed bike with the latest Campagnolo groupset. He also wore Lycra kit, while we remained stubbornly and painfully loyal to wool. One summer's morning, the three of us rode out of London through the suburbs of Tooting, Mitcham and Carshalton, out into the lanes and green fields, beyond Reigate and onto the North Downs. I struggled up the hills and swooped down the descents until, several hours later, we pedalled, kings of the road, into Lewes in Sussex.

It was my first real bike ride. Exhausted, sore and raw, I fell asleep on the train back, a crick in my neck, a pain in my arse and angry tan lines on my legs and arms. We rode back to the flat from the station at twilight, past pubs and pavement tables, oddities, foreign and unexpected.

My woollen cycling jersey, stained white with dried salt from my sweat, sagged from my aching shoulders. I drank endless mugs of hot, sweet tea, then sank into a hot bath. I relived the ride and planned the next route as I fell asleep.

I was already addicted.

AFTER DARK WITH GREG
AND BERNARD

Hovering between my new obsession with cycling and a stalled career, I became fixated with the sense of escape that my bike gave me. I started to have problems sleeping. Too many nights ended prone on the sofa, in front of a TV screen, deep into the small hours, watching videotape of the Tour de France. In the early hours of warm summer nights, I would ride through deserted streets into central London, relishing those stolen hours and imagining the city as my territory, a secret cycling playground. But it exhausted me and after a while, even those nocturnal sorties didn't free me from the guilt of being a disappointment to myself and to others. I'd climb the stairs to the flat, bike on my shoulder, mind buzzing, and seek another escape, watching, over and over, tape of the same race – the 1986 Tour.

That year's race, won by Greg LeMond, was full of intrigue and panache. Both those qualities came in abundance from his team captain Bernard Hinault, who put the hapless LeMond through hell as he reneged on his promise to help him become the first American winner of the Tour, and instead morphed into his most dangerous rival. In the bite-size highlights package on Channel 4, it was enthralling.

It all climaxed in a tense time trial in the hills around Saint-Etienne. By that point LeMond and his team captain were no longer on speaking terms. At the dinner table, their La Vie Claire team was split into two camps: Francophile versus Anglophile. LeMond had become jittery, fearful that his own team was working against him.

LeMond's paranoia was fuelled that day, when he crashed, had problems with his racing shoes and was forced to make a bike change. Bertha LeMond, watching the race with Greg's wife Kathy, leapt off her seat in frustration when she heard of her son's misfortunes. 'Aww, sh . . . *shoot*,' she said, before clasping her hand over her face, mindful of the American camera crew standing alongside.

That's how quaint the Tour was back then, in the years before the old world collided with the new. No effing bad language, no mobile phones or earpiece tactics. Instead, a fraternal hug, a shrug, a smile, a Le Coq Sportif polo shirt and a chilled *vin rouge* at sunset. *Camaraderie et amité* . . .

Greg LeMond can remember all that. He can remember his pioneering ambition, his constant anxiety, the time gaps chalked on a blackboard, the click-clack of typewriters in the press room, the fag-puffing journalists surrounding him, *l'Américain*, on the finish line. He can remember the sheer daring and adventure of the whole damn thing.

There are pictures of LeMond, tanned, youthful, blond, smiling broadly, almost disbelievingly, on the Paris podium in 1989 after he won his second Tour de France by eight seconds from Laurent Fignon. The American is wide-eyed, exultant, near hysterical with joy. A morbid Fignon, ponytail lank with despair, stands beside him, lost for words for once, his face blank with shock, beaten by an American in his home city.

LeMond's success that year remains the narrowest victory margin in the Tour's history.

That win was all the more incredible because he had been close to death following a hunting accident in early 1987. His fight back to Tour de France glory, in the most dramatic finale in the race's history, was American cycling's Hollywood story – until Lance Armstrong came along and beat Greg's three wins and a comeback from being shot with a stunning hand: a return from cancer and seven straight Tour victories.

If LeMond was resentful of Armstrong's success, he had reason to be. As the Armstrong brand took the sports world by storm, with its numerous lucrative extensions, LeMond's groundbreaking achievement was almost forgotten.

Nonetheless, LeMond has always been well liked. The late Rich Carlson, a former editor of mine at *Winning* magazine in the mid 1990s, was naturally a huge fan both of American cycling and of Greg.

'Jeremy, there's something about him,' Rich told me, struggling to find the right words. 'He's . . . well – he's just . . . *folks*,' he said.

Not long afterwards, Rich got sick – very sick – with leukaemia. Greg flew down from Montana to his bedside to see him. The last time I spoke to Rich, down a transatlantic phone line, his disembodied voice tight with pain, he described his illness as a demon on his back. He had been thrilled to see Greg once again, because he knew that he was dying.

Back then, post-LeMond and the late-1980s generation of Andy Hampsten, Steve Bauer, Ron Kiefel and Davis Phinney, North American cycling was, if not in the doldrums, then anxiously awaiting its next Tour de France star. Rich and his magazine badly needed a new hero. Sure, the Armstrong kid was capable of winning a couple of Classics, but he would never have the charm or tactical nous, or the big comeback story, to be able to compete with LeMond.

But we all underestimated him. Rich Carlson, like many others, would have been astounded to have seen Lance win seven consecutive Tours, just as he would have been appalled to see his two cover stars, Armstrong and LeMond, both all-American heroes, at each other's throats.

But because of their polarised stance on doping, Greg LeMond, my TV hero in the flickering light of the midnight hour, and Lance Armstrong, the pivotal figure in my time covering cycling, cannot stand each other.

EPO IS A THREE-LETTER WORD

In 1998, as Lance Armstrong took his first steps towards a full comeback as a professional athlete following his recovery from cancer, the ethical battle in cycling was being tossed around on a sea of acronyms. But it was one three-letter word that took centre stage: EPO.

Armstrong did not ride that summer's Tour, when the house of cards finally collapsed and the full extent of cycling's doping culture was laid bare by the Festina Affair. So crippling were the revelations of systematic doping that the 1998 Tour came close to being abandoned.

Somehow, despite numerous arrests and police raids, walk-outs by disgruntled teams and an unprecedented show of disgust by the French public – which included mooning from the roadside at the suitably ashen-faced Tour boss Jean-Marie Leblanc – the race made it to Paris. The Italian climber Marco Pantani won the Tour, and was hailed as a saviour.

So intrusive were police raids on team vehicles and hotels, it was assumed that all those left racing were competing 'clean'. Surely the French drugs squad had found everything that could be found? By the time the stragglers reached Paris, nobody imagined that Pantani himself might be tainted.

The Tour survived the scandal, but the Festina team was irreparably damaged. Managed by Bruno Roussel, it had started the 1998 race as the world's top-ranked professional team. Their star rider was Frenchman Richard Virenque. He was a perennial favourite, capable of sporadic brilliance on the most coveted and romantic terrain of the Tour, the showpiece mountain stages in the Alps and Pyrenees. With each victory, he would weep tears of joy on live TV. Frenchwomen of a certain age swooned. Rural France, desperate for a new people's hero, took him to its heart.

But Virenque and his Festina teammates were false idols.

The 1998 Tour had started in Dublin. On his way there, while taking a back road to avoid border controls, team *soigneur* Willy Voet was stopped and arrested. Voet was Festina's drugs mule. He was on a road trip across Europe transporting doping products to Ireland.

Taken into police custody, Voet didn't stand up well to interrogation. By the time the peloton returned to France, a fleet of ferries docking at Roscoff in Brittany, he had spilled the beans. Meanwhile, Roussel cracked and told the police that Festina had a medically supervised and systematic doping programme, the products paid for by the riders out of their salaries and prize money. Virenque denied it all – 'Don't turn this into a detective story,' he ranted, ironically, as it turned out – and made a tearful exit from the race when the team were inevitably kicked out. He even published a book, *My Truth*, further rejecting allegations of doping, before finally breaking down in a Lille courtroom and confessing.

1998 had been expected to be a watershed moment: the Tour's great myth, that the peloton competed only on bread and water, had been definitively exposed. The culture of doping was no longer acceptable, neither to the Tour's new audience, nor to the corporate sponsors that were pouring money into the sport. Things had to change.

But they didn't.

When I covered my first Tour de France in 1994, I was aware of the possibility that a minority of cyclists used drugs. Tales of cheating were as old as the Tour itself. I knew that, in the earliest years, riders used to hop between start and finish on the train. I knew about steroids, corticoids and amphetamines. I knew that the most desperate even dabbled with blood transfusions. But I knew little of erythropoietin, to give EPO its full name. Blood doping remained only a distant possibility, the domain of pock-marked, desperate East Europeans. There may have been the odd rogue competitor, but the Tour de France was built on decent, old-fashioned values – in everything I had read, the chivalry, self-sacrifice and honour of the sport shone through. In contrast with world football, the Tour had clung to Corinthian values. Or so, in my naivety, I thought. Yet I soon learned that blood doping had become as common as a yellow card in the Champions League.

The more time I spent in press rooms and team hotels, the more I stood among team cars and on finish lines, the more I chatted across dinner tables where tongues were freed by red wine, the more I understood that doping was everywhere. Cycling had long been a sport of dubious reputation; what I hadn't realised was how inextricably linked it had become to medical technology. Information and gossip about what new products were being used by which rider shot back and forth. And behind it all, was the silence; the unspoken understanding that none of us would give away any trade secrets, because that would be 'spitting in the soup'.

One night, standing outside a Parisian bar with a group of veteran Tour journalists after Miguel Indurain had taken his fifth successive win, conversation revolved around who was taking what and when, how efficiently such a product worked, which rider had been indiscreet, letting slip in a bar somewhere that he had a 'wonder' product that would change his career. 'We have a big problem with EPO,' one of our party said, darkly. By that, he meant rEPO, the artificial version of the naturally produced hormone found in our livers and kidneys. It performs a key function, regulating the manufacture of red blood cells, something which becomes even more important if you're an elite endurance athlete, desperate to find more oxygen during competition.

The more deprived of oxygen we are, the more EPO our

kidneys provide and the more red blood cells zip through our bloodstream carrying oxygen. Hence the attractions for athletes of training at altitude, or sleeping in an altitude tent. Helicopter pilots, one Italian study revealed, would make great endurance athletes – if they weren't flying around the Alps and Dolomites, that is.

When a synthetic form of EPO, called rEPO, was developed in the 1980s to treat kidney failure, and anaemia in cancer and HIV patients, it didn't take long for athletes and their doctors to wake up to the possibilities of enriching the oxygen-carrying capabilities of their blood. Even better, there were no tests within sport to detect its presence.

The potential of rEPO proved particularly seductive in lengthy cycling races, such as the three European tours of France, Italy and Spain, where staving off fatigue and promoting recovery could make the difference between success and failure. In a race as brutal as the Tour, for example, the depletion through fatigue of the red blood cell count, or haematocrit, can be crippling.

No wonder rEPO proved so irresistible to the peloton. It was hugely efficient, undetectable, readily available and, with an estimated twenty per cent improvement in performance, it seemed to guarantee success – or at least survival. It made racing faster, as suddenly everybody in the peloton became an accomplished mountain climber. Overnight, riders who had never won a major race before became uberchampions, their income rising almost as dramatically as their haematocrit. The product endorsements flooded in. They were featured on the covers of Europe's sports newspapers and magazines. After years as also-rans, no marks, they suddenly became stars.

Even though medical supervision was still required, EPO made blood manipulation generally accessible for the first time. And with it, a new generation of sports doctors emerged who openly refused to condemn its use in sport. At the forefront of these was Michele Ferrari, an Italian whose name was to become inextricably linked to that of Lance Armstrong.

There's no doubt that Ferrari − nicknamed 'Schumi' after Formula 1 legend Michael Schumacher − helps his clients go faster. But he is expensive and only the best-paid riders can afford him. Ferrari, who is still actively working with several leading riders, maintains that all his advice is ethical, but in 1994, challenged by French newspaper *L'Equipe* about EPO use, he scoffed at concerns over blood doping, in an exchange which has passed into the folklore of the sport. (It is worth remembering that at this time EPO was not banned, nor was there a test to detect it.)

L'EQUIPE: Do your riders use EPO?
FERRARI: I don't prescribe this stuff, but you can buy EPO in Switzerland without a prescription. If a rider does that, it doesn't scandalise me.
L'EQUIPE: But EPO is dangerous − ten Dutch riders have died in the last few years.
FERRARI: EPO is not dangerous: it's the abuse of EPO that is. It's also dangerous to drink ten litres of orange juice . . .

After saying that, Ferrari became something of a pariah. The team he advised at the time, Gewiss, soon dispensed with his services. As concerns over EPO abuse grew, riders became discreet over their contact with him. He stayed clear of the major races yet hovered unseen in the background of the sport, maintaining his big-name clients.

But despite the warnings of the European press, EPO use in cycling became rampant. It was, and remains, a wonder drug. It is easily available, portable and user-friendly. It achieves results. But there are dangers.

The tales of riders, haematocrit levels soaring, blood thick as sludge, being woken during the night by panicking team staff to prevent cardiac arrests, have become cycling's urban myths. Most journalists have a story of the night they stayed in the Team X hotel and were disturbed in the early hours by slamming doors, panicked voices and the steady whirr of riders training on stationary bikes in their bedrooms, battling to speed their circulation.

They were the lucky ones; some of the others didn't wake up in time.

To state the obvious, blood is fluid. Thickening it beyond the heart's tolerance, through overuse of artificial EPO, can prove fatal. It remains impossible to put an exact figure on the number of athletes who have suffered heart failure through their blood being thickened to deadly extremes. But these days, only the most blinkered dispute that EPO use in cycling became endemic and in some cases led to fatalities.

Some European media reports estimate that between 1987 and 1990, up to seventeen Dutch and Belgian cyclists may have died due to their ill-fated dalliance with EPO. It is certain that many more have since experimented and then become regular users. Those riders were the hapless guinea pigs of a doping revolution.

Twenty years on, the use of EPO has become more sophisticated. Now smaller and more regular doses – known as 'microdosing' – are in vogue. 'Artificial boosting of haematocrit levels a week or more before a race can be maintained by microdosing with EPO three times a week – and still go undetected,' says Michel Audran, a Montpellier-based doping expert.

Faced with this tidal wave of blood doping, with Ferrari's ambivalence over the dangers of EPO, and with growing fears over the riders' health, what did the UCI do?

Until the 1998 Festina Affair provided irrefutable evidence of widespread EPO use, the UCI remained in denial. Cycling, like other sports, had been desperately in need of a definitive EPO test. But at the same time, the development of a successful test could have proved a commercial disaster for a sport that was enjoying a global boom in popularity. If most riders had mastered the use of EPO, a flurry of high-profile positives would have been a public relations nightmare.

How many riders would be caught and how well known would they be? What would be the repercussions legally? What would this do both to corporate and public support of cycling? Would the sponsors cut and run? Faced with this dilemma, the UCI froze in the headlights and opted for a fudge.

In 1997, the UCI introduced blood 'health checks'. In an attempt to end the rampant abuse of EPO, a fifty per cent haematocrit level was imposed and early morning blood testing introduced. For most observers, there was a palpable sense of relief. But the riders, supposedly behind the test's introduction, were more ambivalent: the UCI's visiting medical team was quickly nicknamed 'the vampires'.

The 'health checks' were not a doping test – EPO itself was still undetectable – although it was clear that those with haematocrit levels beyond that magic and seemingly arbitrary figure of fifty per cent would be under intense suspicion. There was no punishment for a failed test; merely a two-week suspension from racing, to 'protect the rider's health'. Once back under the fifty per cent threshold, riders were allowed to resume their careers.

But the suspicion grew that the fifty per cent limit was in fact a tacit legalisation of EPO use, although this suggestion has been vehemently denied by UCI presidents Hein Verbruggen and his successor, Pat McQuaid. It's clear that those with naturally high haematocrit, say of forty-six or forty-seven per cent, have a significant natural advantage over athletes with lower haematocrit. With the fifty per cent limit in place, those with naturally lower haematocrit levels – sometimes as little as thirty-six per cent – now had free rein to top up their red blood cell count and to overcome their natural inferiority. Thus donkeys became thoroughbreds. Everybody could be champion for a day. Unwittingly a level playing field was created, though perhaps not of the kind that the UCI intended. Verbruggen, however, considers this analysis to be 'bullshit'.

In fact, the UCI went to court to defend their reputation after the Festina Affair. They were awarded one euro in damages, but, McQuaid says, the ruling 'stated that the UCI couldn't have done any more to inform the riders of the dangers of doping'.

Yet many experts disagree. Mario Cazzola, of the University of Pavia School of Medicine's Haematology Division, believes that the UCI's 'health check' was inherently flawed. The UCI had based their fifty per cent limit on the results of tests carried out in competition during the Tour of Romandie. However, Cazzola suggests that the baseline for the 'health check' should have been established through out-of-competition testing. Out-of-competition haematocrit – when athletes are not suffering the strain of intense competition – should be *higher* than in-competition haematocrit, when fatigue takes its toll on the red blood cell level. The results of the in-competition 'health checks' revealed that many of the riders seemed to have a surprisingly high haematocrit level of forty-nine per cent – some three per cent higher than the figure the UCI itself deemed 'average'. Even so, the UCI's suspicions were not aroused and they held to the planned fifty per cent limit. Perhaps, given the commercial growth of the sport and the pressure from teams and riders to not undermine them, this limit was no surprise. At fifty per cent, everybody was a winner; the UCI showed that it was getting tough – and the riders could still dose up on EPO.

Cazzola believes that the fifty per cent limit is an inducement for athletes to 'top up' their blood through micro-dosing without risk of detection: 'This is the only explanation I can provide for the elevated haematocrit values frequently found in some professional athletes. Haematocrit levels greater than forty-seven per cent are found in only one or two out of a hundred elite soccer players.

'Upper limits generate aberrant beliefs in athletes: doping is no longer taking rEPO but instead having haematocrit levels greater than the upper limit. Abusing rEPO and having haematocrit values below fifty per cent is felt by some athletes to be fully normal behaviour.'

For Cazzola, blood doping is 'a betrayal of the Hippocratic oath for the physicians who are involved in it. Sport is intended to improve people's health – doping worsens it.' But as the money kept coming in and the Tour's global audience grew, nobody in cycling seemed to be listening.

THE BOTTOM LINE

August 1993, Leeds, Yorkshire. Nearly six months after shattering my knee in Battersea.

My big break. The Leeds Hilton hotel. My first interview, my first 'sold' story. I hobbled through the lobby.

'I am here to see Lance Armstrong,' I announced grandly to the receptionist, leaning on my stick. Her expression was blank.

'Who?' she said.

'Armstrong, Lance Armstrong. He's a cyclist – the Motorola team. Can you, erm, give me his room number . . . please?'

This was my first mistake.

You don't prowl the hotel corridors, you wait in reception. You don't knock, uninvited, on a professional cyclist's bedroom door. You don't disturb their afternoon nap after a hard morning's training.

But, back then, I didn't know that. I went up in the lift. I prowled the corridors, hobbling through the shadows until I found the right door. I took a deep breath, and knocked once, firmly.

No response. I knocked again, harder. And that was how I woke him up. The door was snatched open.

There he stood, all Texan testosterone. Jaw jutting, barrel-chested, frowning, narrowed eyes, clad in white T-shirt and jogging pants, unsmiling – pissed at me already. And I hadn't even opened my mouth.

I stammered through an introduction. He stared at me.

'*Yeah . . .?*' he growled. 'I'm sleeping. Wait downstairs . . .' And the door slammed shut before I could apologise.

I hobbled back through the shadows to the lift, muttering,

'Idiot. *Git.* Blown it, *blown it* – first chance and you've blown it.' I sat in the lobby, despondent, wondering whether it was actually worth waiting, checking my watch and the Leeds to London train times, over and over.

An hour or so later, he strolled out of the lift, chewing gum, wearing a baseball cap, clutching his phone. He even smiled when we shook hands. Everything I'd read about him said he was brash, outspoken, arrogant; very much from the wrong side of the tracks. But it was the softer, more charming Lance who I met that day.

We sat down and talked for about forty-five minutes. He listened thoughtfully to each question. He was dry, funny and sharp. This, in brief, is what he said.

'I don't study cycling, like some people study art.'

'I don't like Europe at all. I really miss the States. When I go home to Italy, life sucks. I miss Texas.'

'I'm not frightened of anybody or their reputations. I grew up on the ropes and I don't have to take anything from anyone. I don't like being told what to do . . .'

'People always think Texans are tough, but there are a lot of wimpy Texans too – it's a big place . . .'

'I don't let the media pressure or the fans' expectations get to me – I mean we're not U2 and I'm not Bono!'

'Last year in the Tour, I found the Alps just incredibly difficult, harder than I'd expected. After that I realised that it will take me a while to become a Tour contender.'

And . . .

'The bottom line is that I expect to win.'

I thanked him and former British professional Paul Sherwen, then working as Motorola's PR officer. We stood up and shook hands. A photographer took Lance outside to pose for pictures with his bike.

'How do you like your bike to be set up?' asked a journalist.

'Man – I just get on it and *ride*,' Lance said. We all laughed.

Two weeks later, arrogantly, brashly, decisively, Lance won the World Championship road race in Oslo. By a street.

'*The bottom line is that I expect to win.*'

JEEPS AND SHOTGUNS

November 1996. Three years on from the Leeds Hilton.

The taxi swept me away from the airport terminal, picked up speed and joined the freeway heading downtown.

Flatbeds, limousines and jeeps slid past, bumper to bumper, in the outside lane. Alongside the slab of elevated road, football stadiums towered over shopping malls and parking lots.

Through the cab's windscreen I saw shotguns stacked against the rear windows of passing trucks, and read bumper stickers with the ominous warning: 'Don't Mess With Texas'.

This was Austin, Texas. Lance Armstrong's home town.

I checked in to the motel, dropped my bags on the bed, downed a bottle of water, and thumbed through my contact book. Lance in Como, Lance in Santa Barbara, Lance in Nice, Lance in Austin, and finally, Lance at Bill's – his agent Bill Stapleton's office. I called the number and scribbled down the address they gave me. I would have to wait. Then I took a shower, switched on the TV, shut my eyes and slept.

Across town, off another exit from another freeway, somewhere on the edge of the Texas hill country, and very much on the right side of the tracks, Lance Armstrong, pale, bald and scarred, was moving slowly through his luxury home on a gated estate. He had been diagnosed with testicular cancer and had undergone surgery and chemotherapy. He'd agreed to be interviewed. At the time, he had seen only a few journalists, mostly American. French sports paper *L'Equipe*, later to become his nemesis, had already been and gone. I was the only other European presence.

The last time I had seen him had been that summer, first at

the Tour de France and then, in August, at the start of the San Sebastian Classic in northern Spain. He'd quit the Tour with a shrug and a wry grin, as a dark thunderstorm swept over Aix-les-Bains. The news broke over race radio as we arrived at the press room. I turned the car around and headed across country to his team's hotel, anxious to find out what was wrong.

I parked up and waited until he arrived. Eventually a Motorola team car swept up to the front door and he hopped out. I walked with him to his room. After he had showered and changed out of his racing kit, we chatted.

'So what happened?' I asked.

'I don't know,' he said with a troubled frown. 'I just feel . . . *blocked.*'

In Spain, a couple of weeks later, we had talked again. He seemed unsure of himself, and kept his eyes hidden behind his Oakley shades. Something was still wrong – that 'blocked' feeling – but he didn't know what was causing it.

The phone rang, waking me from my jet lag.

Lance would see me at the house on Lake Austin the next morning, but they told me to go easy on him and make sure I didn't wear him out. '*If he looks tired, Jeremy, then you gotta stop the interview.*'

Another grey and humid Texan morning. Another taxi, another freeway exit and then we were driving down suburban streets of clapboarded wraparounds with beaten-up trucks parked in scrappy front yards. Under the oppressive sky, dogs on chains sat morosely under porches.

Then, just as quickly, we were out of town, heading towards the shores of Lake Austin through rolling hills and scrubland.

We skirted a hillside overlooking the lake, and slowed at the entrance to a gated community of modernist houses backing onto the water's edge. Sports cars and jeeps dotted the sweeping driveways. Jet skis growled across the lake in the distance.

I didn't know what to expect. My memories of Lance

Armstrong were of a powerhouse jock of an athlete, aggressive, raging, fuelled by intense competitive desire and a quick wit. I rang the bell and waited.

After an age, he came unsteadily to the door, shrunken, slow, washed out, a baseball cap hiding his hair loss.

He was twenty-five, but he moved like an old man. I was so stunned at his decline that I remember that, yes – I very nearly hugged him. I didn't, which given everything that has happened since, may have been for the best. But an arm instinctively went around his shoulder. He registered the shock on my face, straightened himself and smiled.

He walked back into his kitchen and made coffee. Then, for the next hour or so, we sat in his airy lounge with its panoramic views across the lake and high white walls dotted with tasteful contemporary art, talking about cancer. As ever, he was a deceptive interviewee. He can appear relaxed and calm, receptive and open, but every now and then a gesture or a look betrays the tension simmering just below the surface.

He told me about his treatment, about his fear of death, about his hopes for recovery and, with luck, even for a successful comeback.

'I ride for about an hour to an hour and a half as often as I can,' he said. 'But I have to sleep a lot each day. Life's normal apart from sometimes feeling drowsy – and having no hair. But I can take it. As long as I'm alive, that's what matters.'

Cancer, he said, had chosen him.

'Was there anything in your background, your past, to make you susceptible to it?' I asked.

He narrowed his eyes and gave me a stare that was later to become known as 'The Look'.

'A couple of other people have said that and it pisses me off,' he growled. What did he mean? I was baffled.

'Well, erm, I meant in your family history – your mother, your father – if there was any hereditary reason . . .' His face relaxed. It was the only wrong note of the meeting.

Only later, when I read that connections had been made by some between testicular cancer and doping, did I understand his response. But I remained baffled – did he really think that I had flown halfway across the world to make a ham-fisted accusation of doping-induced cancer, even as he endured full-blown chemotherapy?

Kevin, the photographer, finished shooting, packed up his kit and left. Lance relaxed a little more. The physical impact of his illness had made him self-conscious in front of the camera. Relieved, he lifted off his cap and ran his hand over his bald head.

I saw the two angry crescent scars, like ring pulls on a beer can, on the top of his scalp. These were the remnants of surgery on the lesions to his brain. He yawned and rubbed his eyes wearily.

It was time to go.

SOME KIND OF SUPERSTAR, PART ONE

March 1999, the south of France, the final weekend of the Paris-Nice stage race, four months before Lance Armstrong's first and wholly unexpected Tour de France victory.

In the lobby of a hotel in Sisteron, after a day spent racing through the hills of the Vaucluse and Drome, he sprawls across an armchair.

Lance has recovered from cancer. He is not tired any more. He has hair, eyebrows, muscles again. He has a new all-American sponsor, US Postal Service, a team built to serve him, and a very ambitious new team manager, Johan Bruyneel.

And, he has his attitude back.

'Man, the *fuckin'* French,' he says. 'They're so . . .' Unable to find the right words, the sentence trails off, his contempt hanging in the air.

We were discussing the details of a film we were about to make together to coincide with the launch of *procycling* magazine, and to publicise the work of his cancer charity, the Lance Armstrong Foundation. The following Monday we were planning to shoot footage at Lance's house in Nice.

I was one of *procycling*'s launch editors. We didn't have much money but we wanted to make a big statement for our second issue by giving away the film. Nine months after the catastrophe of the Festina doping scandal at the 1998 Tour, the search for a fresh start seemed to be encapsulated by Lance's comeback.

The builders – the 'fuckin' French' builders, that is – should have been long gone by now, Lance said. But being French, they weren't. So we would have to film around them. It might be inconvenient, noisy and distracting, but Lance wasn't going to send them away.

I sipped my coffee. We ran through the agreed schedule one more time. The footage had to be shot in one day. I was aware that he could, just possibly, change his mind at the last moment, that a chorus of drills, hammering and cursing – in Provençal and Texan – might punctuate the soundtrack, but then, like many others, I was learning not to argue with Lance.

When the film crew arrived on the race, there was genuine amusement in the press room. 'Why are you wasting your time making a film about Armstrong?' a Belgian colleague sneered. 'He's finished!'

Ah, but they were all wrong. They had underestimated him. This was Lance The Avenger, back from cancer, lean, focussed, brooding, ruthless, driven to succeed at all costs. He raced anonymously in Paris-Nice, working for his teammates, his eyes on a far bigger prize at the height of the French summer. His dark hair was cropped close, emphasising his new intensity and his high, more pronounced cheekbones. He didn't talk – he *growled*.

At nine-thirty the following Monday, clutching the tattered Michelin 245 that he'd scribbled his address on, we tumbled out of a people carrier outside Lance's villa, high on that *Niçois* hillside. Kids screeched in a nearby playground. I rang the bell. The gate buzzed open and we climbed a set of steps onto the terrace with its panoramic view of the city, the Mediterranean coast and away to the right, the Provençal Alps, where Armstrong had been honing his form.

He and his wife Kristin appeared, cradling mugs of coffee. The French and their inadequacies were still playing on his mind. Despite the noise, he again insisted that the builders carried on working in the house even as we filmed an interview with him beside the pool.

'If they go, they'll never come back,' he said, giving me The Look – his 'this is not up for discussion' stare. *So get used to it . . .*

A little after ten, Kevin Livingston, his US Postal Service teammate, arrived on his bike and in kit, ready for training.

'Late again,' tutted Armstrong, clearly the boss in this relationship.

Livingston offered his excuses, and Lance headed upstairs, reappearing in team kit a few moments later. We trooped down the steps from the terrace and back out through the gate. Armstrong swung open his garage doors, pulled a Trek road bike off the rack and slipped into his racing shoes.

Two minutes later we were crammed back into the van, speeding after them through tight suburban bends as they dropped down from the villa to the foot of the Col d'Eze climb. They swung right and immediately began to ride up the hill, side by side, chatting. Armstrong's style was all latent power, Livingston lighter and more elegant on the pedals, yet somehow less threatening.

A kid on a scooter buzzed past, deliberately close – and far too close for Armstrong's liking. He flew into a rage, yelling abuse and bunching his fist as the scooter moved ahead on the incline and disappeared around a bend.

'*Man, the fuckin' French . . .*'

As they rode on, we overtook them, the back doors of the van wide open, Tony the cameraman suspended over the bumper by bungee cords, filming them as they climbed.

Even now, after all these years, I can remember clearly that on that beautiful March morning Armstrong looked better than I had ever seen him on steep gradients. He was a new rider; as powerful as ever, yet more fluent, and infinitely more at ease. There was an effortlessness to his riding style: the rocking muscularity, the fight against pain, had gone from his climbing.

At the top, in Eze village, we pulled over and filmed as they ordered coffees.

'They shot some of that movie *Ronin* here,' Lance said. But he didn't like stopping. 'I don't wanna catch cold,' he said.

Prompted by Lance, Livingston hurriedly slurped back his coffee and got to his feet.

Quickly, we shot more staged footage, Lance riding back and forth, sprinting at the camera. Then, half a dozen takes later, they were away, flying back down the Col d'Eze with the van, doors swinging open, careering through the bends in pursuit. Tony, snapped this way and that by the bungee cords, howled in protest. Near the bottom we finally sped past and got the shot we wanted – of Armstrong The Avenger, revelling in his renewed athleticism and power, speeding into Nice. We'd been scheduled to spend the whole day filming, but when Lance got back to the villa his mind was elsewhere. 'Come back at two,' he said.

That afternoon, despite the comings and goings of the builder, we shot an interview focussing on Lance's comeback. If the story had become a little familiar now, the depth of his bitterness against those who had written him off still surprised me. He was not in the mood to forgive those who'd spurned him.

'I just keep a list, a mental list, and if I ever get the opportunity . . . I'm gonna pull out that list,' he growled, brow knotted.

'*Jeez*,' I thought as we packed up, 'that's one list I would never want to be on.'

By July 1999, four months on from that breakneck day of shooting, Lance was hot news.

The lobby of the cavernous Westotel on the outskirts of Nantes in western France, was crowded with TV and radio crews, hoping for a glimpse of the new Tour de France leader. I snuck past them, wandering into the deserted dining room – and got lucky. Sitting alone at a round table scattered with the debris of his teammates' breakfast, was the new King of Cycling.

Lance looked up. 'Jeremy! Sit down . . .'

'You sure?' I asked. 'I don't want to interrupt.'

'Hey – you're my friend . . .' he said.

I congratulated him on his win in the Tour prologue and we

chatted and drank coffee together. Photographer Rob Lampard fired off some frames.

In the stage winner's press conference the night before, I'd asked him how he'd coped with the media frenzy surrounding the Tour, eleven months after the Festina Affair. 'Frenzy? About what?' he'd responded, disingenuously.

'So what was all that about then?' I asked him as he poured another coffee.

'Aww, I was just fuckin' with ya,' he grinned.

Finally, he stretched, eased himself out of his chair and we strolled back together to his room.

'Kristin's pregnant,' he told me as we walked.

We had talked about IVF treatment over email. It turned out to be common ground. All the same, I was stunned by their immediate success.

'God, Lance – your life's turning into a fairy tale,' I said.

We talked about defending the yellow jersey and about how far he'd come since I'd seen him in Texas, suffering through chemo, barely able to walk to the door of his house. We didn't talk about the prospect of him winning the Tour de France. That was unthinkable.

'This is it,' he said as we reached the door of his room.

American professional Frankie Andreu rode in the 1999 Tour de France as a valued domestique, *helping his old friend Lance Armstrong to an amazing victory.*

Seven years later, Frankie was at home in Michigan, tidying up his kids' playroom, when, in his deep, calm baritone, he told me how he'd used EPO in preparation for that 1999 Tour.

Like Kevin Livingston, Frankie was one of Armstrong's key supporting teammates that year. He told me he had used EPO only a handful of times, and then only in training, but also that it had improved his performance on the Tour by about twenty per cent. That was enough to ensure he became part of the Armstrong legend.

'I knew what I was doing was wrong, but I had been getting my butt kicked for ten years,' he said. 'I was fine with that — even though I knew I'd get on the start line and wasn't going to win. But then I cracked and got tired of putting up with that. So I did it. But I didn't feel totally guilty about it, because everybody else I was competing against seemed to be doing it.'

As he spoke, in my mind's eye I saw him on the same finish lines that I had stood on, high-fiving with Lance during the good times. It was hard to believe that it was really him, revealing his use of EPO while riding for Lance. Frankie had always seemed a made guy . . . one of the goodfellas.

'Crankie' Frankie, Lance's flatmate in Como during the pioneering 'Euro-dog' days at the Motorola team, and buddy to Max Sciandri, Sean Yates, George Hincapie; Frankie, standing alongside Lance, red-eyed and tearful in his black armband when Motorola's Fabio Casartelli

was killed during the 1995 Tour; Frankie, at Armstrong's bedside when he underwent intensive chemotherapy – he had been through so much with Lance.

How could Frankie have gone over to the other side?

A BOARDROOM IN MAYFAIR

July, 2001. I am walking down Park Lane with Greg LeMond on our way to lunch with a major international oil company to discuss the multimillion-pound sponsorship of a new cycling team and Greg is recounting the tale of his worries about Lance and his spat with Hinault and, yes, I'm listening, but I am also remembering all those late nights watching Greg racing and thinking this is a bit like that Talking Heads song with the 'And you might ask yourself: How did I get here?' line.

Greg is heavier these days than he was, frozen in time on that flickering TV screen in 1986. His hair is greying rather than blond. His face is more sombre and less open than that of the prodigious kid in the yellow jersey. But I can still picture him on Alpe d'Huez, side by side with Hinault, two genuine legends of the Tour, untainted by the suspicion that has dogged every Tour winner since his retirement.

And now, here I am, hoping that, maybe, we might do business together.

In the spring of 2001, an email had dropped into my inbox saying 'I've got £18 million to spend on sponsoring a cycling team. Do you have any contacts who could help me with this?'

I didn't get emails like this every day, and it has to be said that cycling does attract its share of eccentrics. This, however, wasn't one of them.

His name was Jon, and the multinational oil company he worked for wanted to develop a more eco-friendly global image. Bicycle racing seemed to be an ideal vehicle for this.

I took him seriously. We met for coffee. He told me that the plan needed an internationally renowned figurehead who could deliver. I had Greg LeMond's business card in my wallet. Last time we'd met, he'd expressed an interest in trying to put a team together. So I sent Greg an email.

LeMond, who spent much of his time hidden away on his ranch in Montana, was just resurfacing after an ill-fated venture with an American team. He had supplied his own branded bikes to the Mercury-Viatel team, led by a young and enthusiastic former mountain-biking dude called Floyd Landis and managed by the inimitable John Wordin.

Wordin was a gung-ho character, a lean and intense over-competitive dad, lacking in the diplomacy required to gain acceptance on the European scene. At times, his closest sporting relative appeared to be Brian Glover's deranged PE teacher in *Kes*. Wordin, a man apparently battling a midlife crisis, trained with his riders during the day and then fought to balance the books in the evening. Mercury-Viatel's early promise was short-lived, but the eagle-eyed saw that the raw and rebellious Landis was Mercury's star talent; ironically when the team that rode LeMond bikes collapsed in financial disarray, Landis was snapped up by US Postal as a support rider and understudy to Lance Armstrong.

The disintegration of Mercury meant that LeMond's name was once again absent from the European scene – except for when some journo asked him about Lance. That always made the French press twitch with anticipation, especially when Greg told David Walsh of the *Sunday Times*, as Lance homed in on Tour victory number three, that he was 'disappointed' in Lance's relationship with Michele Ferrari. Many wrote his words off as sour grapes – Lance's third victory had equalled Greg's career haul – but that comment began a bitter feud with Armstrong which continues to this day.

When we met, Greg's disenchantment with the peloton was palpable, yet he still wanted to stay in the industry. He believed change was possible. At lunch, we ate well with Jon and his colleagues from the major multinational in a wood-panelled dining room overlooking Hyde Park. LeMond was charming and effusive and hid his disillusion well. But when, over coffee and petits fours, they asked him directly if he could run a team that was clean and still win, his expression darkened.

'I wouldn't want to run a team that wasn't clean,' he answered.

Despite those anxieties, negotiations continued, finally to peter out a few months later. As it transpired, Greg would have other issues to deal with. Soon after he got back from our meeting in London the war between Armstrong and LeMond began in earnest.

A BRUTAL BEAUTY

Like most Italians, Michele Ferrari grew up steeped in the love of cycling. In truth, it was impossible for him to avoid it. If football is integral to British culture, then cycling is just as deeply embedded in the Italian psyche. The great Italian races – Milan-San Remo, the Giro d'Italia, the Tour of Lombardy – are all part of the rhythm of the year, demanding as much coverage in the sports pages as the Champions League or Serie A.

To Italians, sport is about aesthetics, and cycling is about the beauty of a man in union with his machine. It is an obsessive relationship, verging on homoeroticism, fuelled by a century-old tradition, that is encapsulated early every summer at the Giro, where the *tifosi* gather, their camper vans clinging to the mountain sides.

They dot the high passes of the Alps, Apennines and Dolomites, pointing the way to the summits from the valley floor. Ageing, salami-touting, mahogany-skinned couples line the roadside, half-cut on *vino rosso*, wet-eyed and dreaming of past heroes: Coppi and Bartali, Gimondi and Moser, Bugno and Pantani.

The old men emerge from the shade of their camper vans as the *gruppo* pedals through the bends far below and climbs steadily nearer. Lovingly, they unfurl their flags and banners, taking care to choose their spot, ready to run alongside their young heroes, the olive-skinned, brown-eyed, beautiful ones: the Italians.

But recently they have suffered. The Italian cycling scene has long been obsessed with romance, panache and machismo; but the dark side of that obsession, a long-standing fascination with performance enhancement, has been laid bare by a series of high-profile scandals. The most painful one of all left the Italian peninsula in a state of trauma and self-loathing.

Marco Pantani's demented and drug-addled death in a lonely hotel room left a nation in tears. He had been their most beautiful son, a Giro and Tour winner, a heroic gimp in the mountains of Europe, a charismatic but vulnerable athlete who achieved a state of grace and beauty when he sped up the high passes, beyond the reach of his rivals. Pantani was such an explosive mountain climber that he once even brought Lance Armstrong to his knees.

Pantani saw himself as an artiste, a mystic, a guru of the mountains. He developed a habit of talking about himself grandiosely in the third person. He denigrated the scientific methods of others, portraying himself as a rider of whimsy and inspiration, racing on feel and instinct. He railed against the homogenisation of sporting champions, the dour efficiency of automatons such as Jan Ullrich and 'Robocop' Armstrong.

And, fittingly for such a romantic, he died on St Valentine's Day, 2004.

I can remember where I was. We were back from dinner, half watching the news on the BBC, when Pantani's face appeared and the newsreader blandly announced, before telling us to look away now if we didn't want to spoil the suspense of *Match of the Day*, that Marco Pantani, the Italian cyclist, winner of the 1998 Tour de France, was dead.

At least he pronounced his name correctly.

Pantani had died, alone, in an out-of-season beach resort on the Adriatic, a jabbering Viagra-fuelled crack and cocaine freak, lying in a pool of his own blood. He had barricaded himself into his wrecked hotel room, before apparently embarking on one final pharmaceutical orgy.

His full and lengthy decline as an athlete and human being

is charted in Matt Rendell's admirable *The Death of Marco Pantani*, a near-definitive account of a doper's fall from grace and an alarming insight into the darker intricacies of Italian sport. Rendell's book makes for grim reading. God knows how those who profited from Pantani's success and his endless comebacks make sense of his sordid end and their part in his tragic life – and in his gruesome death.

Pantani's death was cycling's Diana moment. But, as Rendell noted, he had been dying for a long time. His was the final betrayal, the moment when many in Italy cried real tears, because cycling had used and abused him, because of collective guilt over his fate and because there had been something so child-like and vulnerable about him when he had first charmed the sporting world.

His unpredictable and volatile nature – he was as likely to be brought crashing down by a stray cat as he was to seal a spec-tacular win – and his defiant *Italianness* ensured his iconic appeal. Once, on a freezing New Year's Day in Flagstaff, Arizona, I walked through the door of a local coffee shop and came face to face with a life-size poster of Marco, staring insolently back at me from behind the Gaggia coffee machine.

Compared to the beefcake champions he challenged – Miguel Indurain, Ullrich, Armstrong – he seemed fragile and under-prepared. His persona flew in the face of the increasingly predictable corporate control of sport. His neuroses and frailties, his impish riding style, his ability to overcome insurmountable odds, appealed to Everyman.

Ten years before Pantani died, I had followed the 1994 Giro, the race in which he first made his mark. At that time, he was naive and awkward, hardly cool, yet Italians were in a feverish state about their new star. He was spindly, balding as opposed to shaven-headed, lopsided, but suddenly brilliant and beautiful in the steepest climbs. He intoxicated his compatriots, sating their need for sporting success achieved with flair and sensuality.

Five years later, he had changed. He wore earrings and

bandanas, was locked in an on-off relationship with a former night club dancer, had become self-destructive and was apparently already overfamiliar with cocaine. Yet only the previous year, in 1998, he had been hailed as cycling's saviour, the 'divine' Marco, redeeming a Tour tainted by the Festina Affair.

That July, when Pantani skipped away towards the highest peaks and final victory, leaving Ullrich, the churning one-paced diesel far behind, he took the hopes of millions with him. But it was an illusion, another stinging betrayal. Within a year, belief in Pantani had been dramatically extinguished. He was evicted from the 1999 Giro on the cusp of final victory. He'd failed the UCI's haematocrit health check, his blood level – analysed no less than eight times – hovering between fifty-two and fifty-three per cent. This did not definitively prove that he had artificially boosted his red blood cell count, but it didn't matter. In the chaotic moments that followed, Pantani was destroyed. He was no longer an innocent. The ensuing scandal broke him, both as a man and as an athlete.

Incredibly, it seems certain that he was a junkie when he rode his final Giro d'Italia in 2003. Cocaine, EPO, crack, Viagra – they all gave him what he craved: success, money, affection, love and power.

Pantani's death was both symptomatic of, and the inevitable culmination of, the unchecked excesses of Italian cycling. His greatest successes came at the very zenith of the EPO years, in the mid to late 1990s. It seems logical to believe that his use of recreational drugs and his subsequent addiction problem was fuelled by his apparent familiarity with doping products in his professional life.

This is the darkest corner of his death, the no-go zone. In the painful aftermath of his death, it was easier for those who knew him to portray him as an unreachable cocaine freak, a wilful drug addict bent on self-destruction, than to ask how he got there and who in cycling held his hand, whispering encouragement, as he travelled down that path.

How could a junkie have competed in three-week stage races, existed within the cycling bubble, without being seen for what he was? For all the tears, Pantani's death was hardly a surprise to anyone who knew him well, yet how he was allowed to go to his death remains a mystery. This was cycling's law of silence as a funeral shroud.

By the end of his life, Pantani's identity, as a human being and as an athlete, was dictated by drugs. He was a work of fiction, unable to realise his true worth, robbed of self-knowledge by the institutionalised doping that surrounded him and to which he'd surrendered himself. Pantani, the mountain guru, the self-styled 'Pirate', the artiste who spurned science and who wore his heart on his sleeve, was as brutalised and cynical, as steeped in self-deception, as any of his peers. Pantani was a flag-bearer for the riders of what became known as Generation EPO, an elite class of cheats that included many of the highest earners of the time. Some of them could handle the day-to-day doping rituals – others, like Pantani, couldn't.

One of those who could handle it and who used it to his advantage, was Bjarne Riis. The Dane was one of a growing number of riders who headed to the heartlands of Lombardy and Tuscany. Many of them, after years of anonymity and isolation, were hungry for success; riding for Italian teams soon sated their appetite. To achieve this success they wholly embraced the Italian philosophy of cycling. And because of that, their careers trace a shady path, of too many doctors, too many allegations, too many tales of soaring haematocrit – and in Riis' case, a banal confession, ten years after the event, of everyday doping to win the Tour de France.

THE TROUBLE WITH BJARNE

In the lobby of an Italian hotel, Bjarne Riis looks through me as if he has never clapped eyes on me before, despite the fact that we have met on numerous occasions.

This is his defence mechanism, perhaps a vestige of an awkward adolescence, a childhood in a broken home; on the other hand he could just be rude. The thing is, with Bjarne, you can never quite tell.

Over the years, partly by accident, partly by design, Riis has cultivated an air of mystery. He could be a deeply complex man, imbued with near-mystical, quasi-shamanic motivational abilities; or a charlatan, cycling's idiot savant who has made a virtue out of saying little, perhaps simply because he has little to say – and plenty to hide.

Either way, he has a strangely compelling charisma and, in his second career as founder and guiding light of the CSC team, he has been phenomenally successful. Riis has an impressive work ethic and an eye for detail. His riders vouch for his guru-like qualities and for his close-knit relationships with his staff. He is serious and studious and takes his team into the Scandinavian wilderness each winter for military-style training camps. He has rekindled the careers and ambitions of Laurent Jalabert, Bobby Julich, Ivan Basso, Tyler Hamilton and Jorg Jaksche, among others.

He has always taken a paternal interest in his riders, teaching a timid Basso first how to swim and then how to win. As a team, CSC have often enjoyed long winning streaks, when they seem unbeatable. But despite that, when it matters most, Riis has often been frustrated. For years, Armstrong and Bruyneel always held the upper hand at the Tour; then, his stars – Basso, Hamilton and Jaksche – all became embroiled in doping scandals during their careers. All of which led us back to Bjarne and to what really lies behind his reclusive nature.

Bjarne had become weary of those nagging worries, ground down by the constant questioning that had dogged him for much of his career.

Even before he confessed to doping, he wanted to move things on, protesting that he couldn't watch his riders 'twenty-four hours a day' and that he believed in clean sport. He has tried hard to build bridges, but he still has a difficult relationship with the Danish media; this uneasiness stretches back to the evening in 1998 when he replied to a Danish TV journalist's question on his own use of drugs with the ambivalent 'I have never tested positive.'

That pressure has eased since 2007, when he finally admitted to EPO use. Since then, Riis has become a virtual recluse, alienated by the sport and making only brief appearances at races, even though he remains the CSC team's key figure. This must have been difficult for somebody with such a quietly controlling personality.

When he first became a professional cyclist, nobody paid much attention to Bjarne Riis. Perhaps it was the diffidence, which often came across as crippling shyness, and the monosyllabic conversation. Even his peers were dismissive of him. 'Beaten by a guy like Riis!' hissed Max Sciandri in horror, after the Dane outsprinted him to steal a rare win.

Like others, I have underestimated Riis, even though I have known him since 1994. Two memories stick in my mind: first, a painfully whispered interview in Pau, halfway through that summer's Tour, which he rode for the Gewiss team. That evening, despite his growing reputation, I was the only journalist interested in talking to him. We sat, uninterrupted, in the lobby of the Ibis hotel, his cathedral dome of a bald pate soaring above me, the pauses between us yawning chasms in the warm evening air. Two days later he won an up-for-grabs stage in the French Midi town of Albi. '*Félicitations*,' said a French journalist wryly. 'You 'ave a scoop . . .'

Then, stuck in traffic on my way to Milan airport on a fading autumnal afternoon at the end of the same season, I saw a different side to him. The final Classic of the year, the Tour of Lombardy, had ended nearby a couple of hours earlier. A Mercedes estate car, bikes on the roof, windows down, music blaring, drew alongside. A group of Gewiss riders were spread across the back seats, laughing and joking. Demob happy, Riis leaned out of the open window, whooping for joy, clutching a bottle of champagne and gulping down mouthfuls of white froth. So much for Nordic cool.

Riis was brought up by his mother in the aftermath of his parents' separation. It took him a long time to come out of his shell. Those who know him say that even as a child, he struggled to find happiness and fulfilment, but as he grew up he rebuilt his relationship with his father through his aptitude for cycling. The young Bjarne's talent won his father's approval.

In the early stages of his racing career, Riis was anonymous, but that changed when he moved to Italy. Before his final seasons with Telekom (later to become T-Mobile) Riis had been one of the senior pros at the Gewiss team, for which Michele Ferrari was the team doctor. Gewiss was like a firework. It exploded onto the scene and dominated racing for two or three seasons. Then, just as quickly, it disappeared. Blink and you missed it.

The team produced a series of stunning performances and spectacular results. They won La Flèche Wallone, one of the toughest Classic races, in an unprecedented manner, after three of their stars turned on their turbos and simply rode away from everybody else. Giorgio Furlan took back-to-back wins in Tirreno-Adriatico and Milan-San Remo, both hugely popular races in Italy; his teammate Evgeni Berzin dominated the 1994 Giro d'Italia.

But aside from Riis' later confession to doping during his period with Gewiss, a dark cloud would follow some of the team's other riders: Berzin was prevented from riding the 2000 Giro after failing a UCI haematocrit test. And, following extensive investigations by Italian journalist Eugenio Capadacqua, reports published in *La Repubblica* and *L'Equipe* in 1999 indicated that both Berzin and Furlan had shown unusually high haematocrit levels in 1995 – the peak period of Gewiss's success. (Both riders' results were over 50 per cent, according to *L'Equipe* – had the UCI's haematocrit test been in place at the time, they would have failed it.) Ferrari's comments had hardly helped: he once claimed that anything that 'can't be found in drug tests isn't doping'. He talked himself out of a job and his riders into trouble.

Greg LeMond described Ferrari as a 'cancer in sport'. But he had his acolytes. If Ferrari was caricatured as cycling's Dr Evil, Luigi Cecchini was his Mini-Me. Riis knew both men, and the connection proved useful in his second career as a team *directeur*. Tyler Hamilton, once CSC's leader and one of Cecchini's clients, described the Italian as his 'second father' after winning an Olympic gold medal at the Athens Games.

Riis has become, by the sport's own standards, one of the wealthiest men in cycling. One estimate puts his career earnings at approximately fifty million kroner, or almost seven million euros, through contracts, endorsements and bonuses. His racing days were ended by injury, for which he pocketed a further two million euros through insurance cover. There are also his earnings from the CSC team sponsorship, through the Riis-Cycling management company, thought to be in the region of five million euros.

Although he now lives in Switzerland, where his children attend an international school, Riis regards Italy, and particularly Lucca, as home ground. He has a property portfolio stretching across Europe, with homes in Italy, Luxembourg, Denmark and Switzerland.

He recently put his home in Denmark on the market for twenty-two million kroner – about three million euros – but, even when the asking price was eventually dropped, was unable to find a buyer. His Italian home, near Lucca, which includes a vineyard, is also thought to be worth about two million euros, as is his house in Switzerland.

A shrewd businessman, there's a story that when new riders joined CSC in 2002, their contract, drawn up by Riis, stipulated that they invested in the downloadable SRM training system, costing approximately three thousand euros a pop. Riis, coincidentally, is Denmark's sole importer of the SRM system.

He is thick-skinned and determined, a hard worker and a survivor. 'Bjarne has to be the best at everything, even if it's just making a cup of coffee,' says Lars Werge, a Danish journalist who knows Riis well. 'Even though he is unassuming, he can be ruthless.'

Yet for all his ambition, one great prize, victory for his own CSC team in the Tour de France, had always eluded him. Time after time, Armstrong stood in his way. But then Bjarne's gaze settled on a diffident but highly gifted young Italian called Ivan Basso. What would it take to turn the underachieving Basso into a contender?

'HE WILL NEVER BE PANTANI . . .'

January 2006. On the slopes of Monte Serra in Italy, Bjarne Riis, the Scandinavian sporting guru, speaks: 'Maybe you should go now,' he tells a British journalist menacingly, halfway up this Tuscan mountainside.

Riis turns on his heel and walks back to his CSC team car. The hapless journalist shrugs, climbs into his car and heads back down the hairpins. If you want to watch Riis training and working his CSC team and staff, it's best to ask nicely first.

Based at an anonymous seaside hotel at the windswept Lido di Camaiore, north of Pisa, CSC – with Lance Armstrong now retired – were expecting 2006 to be their long-awaited break-through year in the Tour. The team were training hard, spending long days out on the road, testing themselves and their equip-ment. The riders had settled into the familiar routine of sleeping, eating, riding. There was little else to occupy them.

The taxi driver who took me from Pisa airport to the hotel got excited when I told him I'd flown in to meet Ivan Basso. 'Basso – a household name! But,' he sighed sadly as we left the autostrada and joined the coast road, 'he will *never* be Pantani.'

CSC were pinning their hopes for 2006 on Basso, who had scaled new heights since joining forces with Riis. The Italian's stock was high and with Armstrong gone, many saw him as a potential Tour de France champion.

The Hotel Caesar had opened specifically to host Basso and the CSC team for a two-week training camp. Good coffee and a lavish buffet were available around the clock. Riis, his family in nearby Lucca beckoning, was said to be missing his kids, so some nights he slept at home.

On the wall of the lobby by the lifts, was a list of the riders' room numbers. As usual, Bobby Julich was paired with Jens Voigt. It is received wisdom in cycling that it is good for morale to share a room, especially with a close friend. Only superstars – Armstrong, Ullrich and here at CSC, Basso – don't share. Near the room list, there was also a list of departure times for visits to an unnamed doctor. CSC was in Tuscany to train – and to be photographed and interviewed. The next morning the riders dutifully stepped out into the icy air for the new season's promotional shots. The same scenario was being repeated in out-of-season resorts all along the horseshoe of the Mediterranean and the locals looked on with jaded expressions as they sped by on their Vespas. One by one, the riders struck a pose, usually against a carefully chosen backdrop of team car or minibus (although on this occasion, the Hotel Caesar's flagpole). They puffed out their weedy chests and smiled determinedly with a look that said, '*Yes! This year will be my best-ever season!*'

Without the tan lines of high summer and the battle scars of competition, the riders looked out of place. Their frighteningly low body fat was no protection against the freezing wind. They shivered like worried whippets as the photographer fiddled with his lenses.

Stuart O'Grady pedalled out into the chill air. 'Bet you love these promo shoots,' I said. '*Oh yeah* – 'specially when it's nice and warm like this,' the Australian responded, the goosebumps rising on his freckled arms.

Next came the team photo. The riders click-clacked through reception in their cleated shoes and perched precariously, all fixed grins, on the edge of the hotel pool. It was very cheesy, a real Eurotrash moment. 'All we need now are shaggy perms,' sneered Brian Nygaard, the team's PR officer.

Pictures taken, they trooped back inside, donned their thermal gear and got ready to leave for training. Ten minutes later, I climbed into the back seat of CSC's mobile management suite, a customised Renault Espace laden with CSC's *directeurs*, seated respectfully just behind team guru, Riis.

'Everybody give me a *boo-yah*,' called the self-consciously zany Dave Zabriskie, reputed to base his every word on the script of *The Big Lebowski*. What did the 'Zee-Man' mean? It didn't matter. A booming, albeit half-hearted, '*Boo-yah*' echoed back, as CSC's riders began to move out of the hotel car park.

Off the leash at last, the riders wove expertly through the Passats, Puntos and Clios that clogged up the streets of Camaiore, and headed inland. Riis watched impassively from the front seat of the Espace. He studied a spreadsheet documenting the test results of the training camp so far and in particular of the previous day's climbing trial. Fourteen of CSC's riders had ridden a timed mountain test within fifty seconds of each other. So early in the season, it was an impressive collective performance.

The kilometres passed. Riis completed his assessments and picked up the CB radio linking the Espace to each rider's earpiece. He spoke calmly in English to them: 'Gentlemen, spin the legs. Transform the power of yesterday into the power of today. Always make sure you keep a good rhythm.'

He turned his gaze back to the results. The riders had so far been tested twice, on different ascents of Monte Serra nearby. The most recent trial was over 6.4 kilometres on what Riis calls 'the climber's side'. Riis still holds the record for the climb, dating from the summer of 1996, the year he won the Tour de France, a victory sealed through doping.

As we headed further inland, there was no doubt who was the CEO of CSC's cycling team. 'We need to evaluate progress,' Bjarne said.

'You remember the watts from Dave?' he said into the CB radio.

'Give me ten minutes. I'll check on the laptop,' replied assistant *directeur* Scott Sunderland from another team car somewhere in the Tuscan countryside.

While he waited, Riis pulled out a handycam, leaned out of the window and began filming the riders ahead of him. 'They like to see it,' he explained. 'It's a record of training. If we say, "Maybe you should move your saddle a little bit," it helps if we can show them why. It's not to prove a point, but if somebody really doesn't agree, then we have the tape to show them . . .'

Sunderland's voice crackled over the CB radio. 'Dave was 459 watts, 187 heart rate and 82 cadence. Ivan was 437 watts, 185 heart rate and 78 cadence.'

Riis considered the information before delivering his verdict. 'Dave will win straight away, but all of them are ready to race. This is the most competitive team we have ever had.'

He spoke into the radio again. 'Three groups, please. Stay in the same three groups.' For a moment, there was a hiatus as riders freewheeled and gaps opened. Then they came together again, as if choosing new partners on the dance floor.

Suddenly, a gap of a hundred metres or so opened between each of the three groups. Then the pace assumed a new intensity. Riis explained that the first group was preparing for the Giro, the second for the Tour, the third for the imminent Spring Classics. They rode on as a biting crosswind pulled at the cypress trees and olive groves.

CSC has some expertise at this. In the past, the team has split races apart by sending the entire team to the front of the field in bad weather, usually driving rain or crosswinds. Riis wanted them race-hardened even before the season begins.

'They have to ride a bit harder, work in the wind a bit harder,' Riis said. 'Technically, it's more demanding and they have to work together more.'

Not all Italians love cycling. The occasional driver overtook, horn blaring, fist raised as the CSC convoy of team cars and hangers-on moved across the Tuscan landscape. The riders ignored it. They pedalled smoothly ahead of us in three uniform groups.

The wind picked up, tugging at their shoulders as they hunched over the handlebars. Dusted with snow, the Apennines loomed large. This, however, was a flat day's training, with the emphasis on speed and fluency. There was to be no cruel assessment on the steep slopes of Monte Serra.

Back in the mobile manager's suite, assistant *directeur* Tristan Hoffman began telling a tale about one of my colleagues.

'This journalist sent me a text in the middle of the night. It said: "Don't let's fight. I loved the sandwich. Can't wait to see you again." So it wakes up my wife and she says, "Who's this from? What sandwich?!" She's seven months pregnant and I've just got home from a trip! So I told her, "Call the guy," but she doesn't believe me and thinks I've got my excuse ready in advance . . .'

Everybody guffawed at Hoffman's misfortune. I laughed uneasily and tried to defuse the situation. 'Well – he's always getting phone numbers mixed up. He's done a similar thing to me . . .'

Riis' face suddenly turned to thunder. 'He did it to you too? *What an asshole!* Can't he use a phone?'

An hour later, the normally impassive Riis finally came to life. He stood grinning like a schoolboy over a new train set, watching proudly as one by one his riders sped down the windswept road from a standing start, in a mock time trial. One by one they came back to the impromptu start and finish line, mouths open in exhaustion, as a delighted Riis slapped them on the back in encouragement. Chilled to the bone, we climbed back into the Espace and headed for the hotel.

It was nearly lunchtime.

Hoffman had sandwiches on his mind again. He reached into the coolbox on the back seat and pulled out a roll, wrapped tightly in foil. 'Looks like *prosciutto crudo*,' he guessed.

'No,' snapped the monotone voice in the front passenger seat. 'It's *prosciutto cotto*,' said Bjarne Riis, correcting him.

Bjarne Riis' career spanned an era of huge cultural changes in cycling, a period in which doping transformed itself from a cottage industry into the currency of success. As a rider, he was first a *domestique* to the last Frenchman capable of winning the Tour, Laurent Fignon. Then he established himself as the guiding light of the Telekom team, and plotted the downfall of Miguel Indurain.

Later, he became a mentor to Ferrari and Cecchini protégés, Evgeni Berzin, Jan Ullrich, Tyler Hamilton and Ivan Basso. As a *directeur sportif*, he was a bitter rival to US Postal's powerbrokers, Armstrong and Bruyneel, during their seven-year dominance of the Tour.

Throughout that period of almost twenty years, Riis has adapted to the needs of his sport. He is a chameleon, able to maintain his footing on shifting sands. He is the professional scene's Everyman, one minute doping himself on an everyday basis, the next manning the ramparts in the battle for clean sport. He has been buffeted by scandal but seems capable of constantly reinventing his place in the sport's hierarchy.

He was a self-appointed peacemaker in the Festina Affair and, nine years later, found himself in the eye of the storm once more, as the fallout from Operacíon Puerto, the 2006 doping investigation in Madrid, settled on his star rider, CSC team leader Ivan Basso.

Following that scandal, Riis instituted radical anti-doping checks within the CSC team and now exhibits an acute understanding of the financial relationship between his sponsor's brand and his team's image. But many find it almost comical that Bjarne Riis is pleading for transparency, accountability and a clean sport.

The man who once responded to a direct question about his own attitude to doping with a smirk and the response 'I have never tested positive' wants us to forget his past. 'Cycling needs me,' he says.

OK, Bjarne, and maybe it was all a long time ago, but these things are not easy to forget.

And so it was that finally, eleven years after his unexpected win in the 1996 Tour de France, Bjarne Riis – as haunted as anyone in cycling by the ghosts of that decade – sat down and confessed.

'I have taken EPO,' he said in a press conference in Copenhagen. 'It was a part of everyday life as a rider.'

There is a clip on YouTube of Bjarne Riis addressing the media in Copenhagen, head bowed, confessing his sins and seeking absolution. Was he a worthy Tour de France winner, somebody asked him. 'No,' he said, 'I am not.'

And once the dam had broken, the truth about Bjarne's EPO habit came pouring out. 'I have taken doping,' Riis said. 'I purchased it myself and I took it myself. I did things that I shouldn't have and I have regretted that ever since. Those were mistakes that I take the full responsibility for and I don't have anyone to blame but myself. I am a lot wiser now, both in my personal and in my professional life.'

But Riis, who admitted doping himself throughout the most successful years of his career, seemed to be in no hurry to return his 1996 yellow jersey. 'I'm proud of my results even though they were not completely honest. I'm coming out today to secure the right future for the sport. My jersey is at home in a cardboard box,' he said. 'They are welcome to come and get it. I have my memories for myself.'

Riis' confession, delivered with humility and gravitas, was received with scepticism and scorn. If the original clip makes dramatic viewing on YouTube, far better value is Team Easy On's subtitled bastardisation of his confession, easily the best of a crop of bitching and vitriolic attacks. Ashen-faced in contrition he may have been, but for people who'd spent more than a decade listening to his lies, now was the time to put the boot in.

Team Easy On's voiceover, straight out of a Dutch brown bar, takes Riis' doping excesses to a surreal conclusion, listing skunk, opium and heroin among his preferences. 'It's funny that you ask about my physical condition,' runs the voiceover, as Riis stares sombrely into the camera, '. . . because my heart *eksploded,* and because of that I had to go to Africa because I have many connections in Congo . . . So I went down to a guy called Pepsi Franck and bought myself a whole new heart . . .'

So much for the myths and legends of the Tour de France: Riis, once feted as a national hero in Denmark, was now an Internet freak, to be ridiculed over and over again. But not everybody in his home nation found it so easy to see the funny side.

Lars Werge, one of Riis' chief tormentors through a decade of suspicion, was vindicated by Riis' admission of guilt. But it left a bitter taste in the Danish sports writer's mouth. 'I was angry that he had been lying for so many years. And it made me angry that he thought, that by telling the truth, it would all somehow be OK. It was like a marketing stunt.'

Werge was not alone in thinking that Riis' motivations were not solely founded on a desire for truth and reconciliation, but also from a need to salvage crumbling relationships with his disenchanted sponsors.

'Some people felt sorry for him and over the next few days a lot of people were interviewed about him,' Werge recalls. 'I said that maybe it would be better if he left cycling. But I was criticised for saying that because people knew that he was in a sport in which it was difficult to tell the truth.'

There was guilt, shame and a little self-pity to be found in Bjarne Riis' statement that day. The vulnerable boy from a broken home, desperate for his father's approval through his achievements as an athlete, was suddenly visible.

'We all make mistakes. I think my biggest mistake was to let my ambition get the better of me,' he said. 'I'm sorry if I've disappointed people. To those for whom I was a hero, I'm sorry. They'll have to find new heroes now.'

Part Two

Positive Thinking

'History repeats itself – the first time as tragedy, the second time as farce.'

Karl Marx

In the wake of the crippling Festina Affair of the 1998 Tour de France, Lance Armstrong's first victory in 1999 was acclaimed as a 'Tour of Renewal'. A new generation of riders – including David Millar – was breaking through. With this influx of youth came a surge of hope that the sleazy habits of the past might finally die out. That optimism did not last long.

The scale of the Festina investigation and the subsequent trial in Lille had revealed the abject failure of the sport to police itself. The UCI took much of the blame, although the governing body's president, Hein Verbruggen, put up a staunch defence. But Verbruggen, guardian both of cycling's ethical well-being and its commercial health, had an obvious conflict of interest.

It became increasingly clear that the UCI's doping controls had become inadequate; instead, the police did their work for them, with a series of raids at races and at the homes of individual riders that further revealed how endemic doping had become. This was precisely how Millar, at the time the reigning world champion and British cycling's golden boy, was caught.

Paradoxically, the period immediately after the Festina Affair was also the moment when things might have changed for the better.

The Pandora's box of secrets had been opened. A new era in a sport notorious for doping might have begun. Another generation of fans and riders might have been spared a great deal of anguish. Yet there was no discussion of what kind of sport professional cycling in the modern era should be. The opportunity to discuss the brutal demands of the racing calendar, the health needs of the riders and the composition of the banned list of doping products slipped away. Instead, doping practices were merely driven further underground.

The moment had been lost: the lid slammed shut again.

Armstrong carried on winning to become the most dominant champion in the history of the sport, creating a tidal wave of wealth in his wake. Without a moment's thought for the consequences, the sport scrambled to make the most of the opportunity. Meanwhile, the UCI, torn between ethics and commerce, froze in the headlights once more as the untapped wealth of the stateside market hove into view. Armstrong and Bill Stapleton had known that, if all the right circumstances combined, Lance could bring unimagined wealth into cycling. Hence the Texan's firm refusal to dirty the sport's image by acknowledging the extent of cycling's doping problem and Verbruggen's insistence on shooting the messenger for the next six years.

'I am sick of the myth of widespread doping,' Armstrong had said as the 2000 Tour began. Yet by the end of 2006, no less than five of his key teammates — Frankie Andreu, Tyler Hamilton, Roberto Heras, Floyd Landis and one other anonymous former US Postal rider — and countless peers and rivals had either tested positive or admitted to doping. The runaway train was still careering down the tracks.

As the authorities across Europe became more actively involved in breaking up doping rings, trust within the sport broke down. Room-mates and best friends gave each other up. A climate of fear and paranoia took hold. Police raids and scandals proliferated, fuelled by an unprecedented development in cycling: the culture of the whistle-blower. The law of silence, the omerta, *appeared to be finally losing its grip.*

In France, the whistle-blower's talisman was Christophe Bassons; in Spain, Jesus Manzano; in the USA, Matt DeCanio and, in Italy, Filippo Simeoni. None of them were afforded any protection by Verbruggen or the UCI and, in what was little more than a witch-hunt, they found themselves ostracised, written off and even threatened, as if their experiences were invalid, their careers expendable. Yet when star riders fell foul of traditional dope tests, they vehemently proclaimed their innocence. In contrast with those such as Millar, whose brutal police interrogation led to a swift admission of guilt, Tyler Hamilton and Floyd Landis called in their lawyers and attacked the credibility of the testing procedures. This only further polarised the sport and created a draining moral maze of acronyms, legalese and technicalities, in which even the most hard-bitten anti-doping campaigner soon became lost.

Supported by lawyers, sponsors and fundraising websites, such as ibelieveintyler.org and floydfairnessfund.com, Hamilton and Landis went on the offensive. As Armstrong's career closed with a seventh successive Tour win in 2005, and a tub-thumping speech exhorting us all to believe in the sport, the omerta clung on.

Still the scandal continued. Riders blamed their federations, the media, French testing procedures, anti-Americanism, the UCI, the IOC, LNDD, WADA, USADA – in short, everybody but themselves . . .

FALLING DOWN

In 1998, David Millar, a fresh-faced second-year professional cyclist from Scotland (via Malta, Hong Kong, London and Biarritz), said: 'When I'm out training and someone shouts "doper", I feel like I want to stop and swing for them. It upsets me to think that people assume every pro is on drugs.'

In 2006, David Millar, making his comeback following a two-year ban after he confessed to using EPO, said: 'I fucked up, I cheated and I have to live with it.' David Millar never failed a drugs test. So what happened?

November, 2003: David Millar, world champion, Tour de France stage winner, Olympic hopeful – and self-confessed dandy – is on the dance floor in a Manchester bar vigorously shaking his bony ass. I observe the scene, perched unsteadily on a wobbling bar stool.

Teenage girls, perhaps more hopeful of a glimpse of Ryan Giggs, Joey Barton or Cristiano Ronaldo, look unimpressed as Millar throws some unfamiliar and decidedly uncool shapes.

We are both, to paraphrase Lance Armstrong's words about David and his love of partying, drunk on our ass.

I had seen David do many things, but I'd never seen him dance before. Through a fog of beer and wine, I watched him duckwalk his spindly frame into a ball, before exploding back to his full height in spasms of exuberance. Like a crop-haired Russell Brand, he shimmied across the floor towards me, unshaven, wide-eyed, gurning dementedly. I lurched back onto my seat and prayed for this breakneck night of excess to end.

"Nother one, Jez?' he bellowed in my ear, as my head slumped further between my shoulders.

David likes a drink. So do I. But this uneven contest was the shipwreck of an interview that started out innocently enough in David's loft apartment. Chris Boardman was also there, and the three of us sat talking, sipping chilled beer as dusk fell over the Pennines. After Boardman had gone home to his wife and kids, I realised too late that I should have followed suit. Instead the evening degenerated into a sad spectacle – at least on my part.

What is it about top athletes that allows them to tie one on and then shake it off the next day? Once, after a night spent celebrating a friend's birthday in his favourite Biarritz bar, we'd followed Millar on a training ride into the Pyrenees, only to bale out after the first mountain pass when the photographer lost his breakfast on the ladder of hairpin bends.

That night in Manchester, deep into his off-season, David was in his cups. I couldn't keep up. So what did I learn from this experience? I think the key message to pass on is never drink with Olympic-level athletes – many of them are also Olympic-level drinkers . . .

I liked David Millar immediately, perhaps because he was so different to other athletes that I had met. He was irreverent, intelligent and funny, with a big smile, angular good looks, and an open nature. He was interested in the world beyond his sport, and beyond The Race.

Even now, four years after he was banned for doping in 2004, I can't help but feel protective of him. Perhaps it's because underneath the 'it's all good' bravado, there remain occasional glimpses of a defensiveness and vulnerability. These days, he's developed a thick skin, having been kicked from pillar to post in the aftermath of his ban.

From our first meeting at the Tour of Switzerland in 1998, it was clear that Millar loved cycling. He had an encyclopaedic knowledge of the sport's recent history. He was seduced by the travel, the glamour, the romance and the danger of the European scene – and, crucially for somebody who had spent a nomadic adolescence, by the same sense of belonging that first reeled me in.

'I love bike racing,' he said. 'I love it when it's really extreme, when it's raining and snowing. Even on days like that, it's your job to finish – even when you've fallen off and are covered in blood, or have broken a bone. That's the ethos of the sport – if you can pedal, you carry on.'

He lived in a small flat amid the faded grandeur of surfer's paradise, Biarritz. Being some distance from the spring circuit of Mediterranean races and lacking a major international airport, it was an odd choice for a professional cyclist. Most riders lived in clusters in towns like Nice or Toulouse. Given his maverick nature, his leaning towards a solitary life and his ambivalence towards the professionalism of his job, it suited Millar well. He became an adopted son, a local hero – '*un vrai Biarrot*'.

In fact, the Atlantic resort, close to the Pyrenees, buzzy, quirky and with good nightlife, was ideal for him, as he cultivated his image as a latter-day English eccentric. After he won his first yellow jersey in the 2000 Tour, the French press christened him '*Le Dandy*'. Millar loved it.

In the autumn evenings, the racing season over, the wind whipping up the Atlantic rollers, he would shut himself away in a restaurant with local hero André Darrigade, a former Tour de France star. Darrigade had become a local newsagent, and Millar would listen, rapt, to stories of the Tour when it was still a dashing Hemingwayesque event for oddballs, rogues and renegades. The influence of past stars such as Darrigade and, to a lesser extent, mythologised characters such as five-time Tour winner Jacques Anquetil, who drank champagne, played poker, had numerous complicated romances and drove fast sports cars – sometimes all on the same night – all shaped Millar's devil-may-care outlook.

Yet when I got to know David better I realised that while he loved the romance of the sport, a part of him increasingly resented the demands it made of him. I could sense his internal conflict and his yearning for a more normal life. At those times, often when he most felt the pressure to achieve success, he was at his most volatile and vulnerable.

When he won the prologue time trial in Futuroscope and took the yellow jersey on his very first day in the Tour, David wept. He hugged his mother Avril, his tears wetting her 'It's Millar Time' T-shirt. One French regional newspaper called him *procycling*'s '*chou-chou*' — *procycling*'s darling.

My darling — and yes, before he fell into the viper's nest, David was.

David Millar liked to train hard and play hard. His first flatmate in Biarritz, fellow British pro Jez Hunt, struggled to keep pace with Millar's demands for challenge and entertainment, both on and off the bike. Another British pro, track-racing veteran Rob Hayles, moved to Biarritz briefly, but was soon exhausted both by his racing schedule and the 24/7 demands of life with Millar.

David was different to the other riders, many of whom had grown up in quiet French towns, or in the backwaters of Switzerland, Spain, Belgium and Italy. He sought acceptance, yet he remained independent and stood out from the crowd. He was middle class and exotic, and try as he might, it showed. His father flew long haul for Cathay Pacific and his mother successfully became CEO of her own business in central London. David could have gone to art school, studied photography or slipped into the easy money of the expat business community in Hong Kong. Instead, he chose to become a professional cyclist, simply for the love of it.

Lance Armstrong, briefly his teammate at Cofidis, was an early professional contact who became a friend. Like David, Lance came from a broken home and like David, he had a difficult, in Lance's case near non-existent, relationship with his father. But where David was vulnerable and inconsistent, Lance was ruthless and raging, both brutalised and brutal.

Their parents' divorce was traumatic for both David and his sister Fran. They spent much of their adolescence flying backwards and forwards between Avril in London and Gordon in Hong Kong, at that time still a playground for middle-class kids. Yet he was rootless after his parents split up, not living in one place or the other, one of those sullen preteens in airports with a label hanging from their neck. Finally, he settled in Maidenhead in Berkshire, where his mother lived.

But Avril worried about her teenage son and encouraged him to make friends. He joined a cycling club and almost immediately won races. Soon he was competing at a high level, both in the UK and abroad. Through all his travels, David had become something of a chameleon. He was eloquent, moody and thoughtful. But he was also a boy racer, a posh lad, a drinker, a ringleader and a good talker, able to walk into a group and quickly find what was needed to fit in. That skill helped him when he first moved to France.

When he arrived at the French-sponsored Cofidis team, another set of expats – Tony Rominger, Lance Armstrong, Bobby Julich and Frankie Andreu – were part of the all-star set-up, although when they left (Armstrong dramatically in exile because of his cancer, Rominger forced to retire, Andreu and Julich to other sponsors) Millar once again found himself isolated.

He had to fit in somehow, so he became an entertainer, the cute lead singer to what had become an anonymous backing band of journeymen professionals. After a couple of early wins, he found himself in demand.

There was the yellow Land Rover he'd driven down to Biarritz – 'so Breeteesh' – the designer labels and the dyed hair. He was soon on the covers of magazines, the peloton's Robbie Williams. Somewhere along the way, as he yearned for acceptance in a world in which he was always likely to be an outsider, David Millar mixed up being a professional cyclist with being in a band.

In 2003, clad in Great Britain's team colours, his hair chopped and bleached, David stood on the podium, eyes closed, listening to 'God Save The Queen' as he celebrated his win in the World Time Trial Championship in Canada. Hours later, he and a group of fellow pros began a forty-eight-hour bender that took him to a suite in the Bellagio and to a wild party that became the talk of the Interbike trade show in Las Vegas.

Dishevelled and red-eyed the morning after, he stumbled late onto the *procycling* stand at Interbike for a meet and greet with the magazine's readers. His tousled state left most of them wondering how on earth he had won a world title in the first place.

As 2003 ended, David appeared to have it all. Paul Smith, thinking of using him as a model. Cofidis were dangling what was in essence, with bonuses, a million-euro contract. He was a world champion who talked of the importance of respect from his peers and saw himself as one of the bosses in the peloton. David's life had become a high octane, high-wire act, fuelled by his charm, energy and opportunism.

But he was living on borrowed time. In June 2004, Millar lost everything. He had never failed a drugs test, but, detained and questioned by the French police and an investigating judge, he admitted that at certain key periods in his career he had doped himself with EPO. The police followed the path to his door opened by the testimonies of Philippe Gaumont, his former Cofidis teammate. In his book *Prisoner of Doping*, Gaumont described his own initial flirtation with drug use and then detailed his subsequent immersion in institutionalised doping. Published in France in 2005, as *Prisonnier du Dopage*, Gaumont talks movingly of Millar, his young British teammate, tormented by his parents' divorce, by his vulnerability, by the expectations placed upon him and by his nomadic lifestyle.

'He was fragile,' Gaumont wrote, as he detailed Millar's excesses, fuelled by the boredom of his hotel room at training camp.

Gaumont described the relationship between Millar and Cofidis team doctor, Jean-Jacques Menuet. 'There was a strong link between them, because of David's difficult childhood,' he wrote. 'I say difficult, but maybe that's not the right word. David's parents had means . . . and, for a cyclist, you could say that he'd had a rare education. He had studied and could have gone to art school, if he hadn't chosen cycling . . . He spent his teenage years left to himself, shuttling between England and Hong Kong. He always gave the impression he had something to prove.'

Gaumont's compassion towards Millar contrasted sharply with David's own description, as the Cofidis scandal grew, of the Frenchman as 'a nutter'.

'I believe,' wrote Gaumont, 'that Millar felt bad about cheating. It gave him a bad conscience, but like many of us, like me at any rate, he no longer knew how to stop. To forget about it all, I saw him take refuge in drugs and medication . . . It's funny but when I look at him, he reminds me of myself. The more the seasons passed, the more he lost his innocence.'

Gaumont's litany of his own chaos, self-abuse and addictive behaviour was unflinching. He was equally unsparing of others. He detailed widespread use of cocaine, ephedrine, Stilnox – plus EPO for racing – and described the curious prudishness of some of his own teammates who were appalled at his post-racing recreational drug use, but blithely encouraged doping in the hunt for results and financial rewards.

When the Cofidis scandal broke in the spring of 2004, Gaumont was the principal whistle-blower, pouring out his trade secrets to investigating judge, Richard Pallain. In March that year as he raced for Cofidis in Paris-Nice, Millar was paranoid, melancholic, defensive. I spoke to him in the start village at Digne-les-Bains. He was dressed up and ready to race, but I could tell that his heart was no longer in it, as if he knew what was coming.

Gaumont, as Millar and others kept telling me, was 'a nutter', a loose cannon who had lost his mind. But as he said it, I could see his anxiety. He rambled on about phone taps and security cameras and my heart sank when, as I stood there in the spring sunshine listening to him, I finally realised that David too, had fallen from grace.

'You're talking about absolute bullshit from this lunatic Philippe Gaumont,' Millar said. 'That's what it is and it's hard to express to people the degree of bullshit this is. Then you see a newspaper listening to him . . .'

And a journalist, Dave, like me, listening to him.

Millar admitted that he liked Philippe Gaumont. 'I got on really well with him,' he said. 'It just baffled me. He's in trouble and he's gone for the guys in the team who'd hurt the team most: the leader and the management.'

Spring turned to early summer. Millar carried on racing, anxious, empty-hearted and fearful, protesting his innocence, blaming the 'nutter'.

Gaumont, meanwhile, carried on talking to the judge.

The clock finally stopped for Millar Time early on a June evening.

David was seated at a table in a Biarritz restaurant with GB team performance director, David Brailsford and his partner. Outside, in the car park, a saloon car slalomed to an abrupt halt.

The French drugs squad had arrived from Paris, Gaumont's testimony to Judge Pallain ringing in their ears. They were on a mission to rein in the excesses of this young foreigner. They marched into the restaurant, stood over the table and ordered Millar to follow them outside.

'We'd had a first sip of wine,' Millar remembers, 'and three guys turned up, showed their badges and said, "David Millar – come with us." They took me out into the car park, took my watch off, my shoelaces, any jewellery I had, my keys and phone. I started speaking in English and asked for a translator . . . and they said, "If you want a translator we'll put the cuffs on you." '

Millar felt a rising sense of dread. 'They were drugs squad. They'd driven down from Paris that day, couldn't find me at first so then, when they finally found me, they were pumped and they were angry. They were treating me like I was a cocaine dealer. They were pretty rough on Dave Brailsford and his girlfriend too, and she was heavily pregnant. They took me back to the apartment. They went in with a gun first, as if somebody was going to hit them with a back wheel, or something. They sat me down and I wasn't allowed to move, while they searched the house. It took them four hours. I said to them, "Why are you here?"'

Millar says he was systematically humiliated. 'They were criticising my lifestyle, using a classic good cop/bad cop thing. It was psychological warfare. The bad cop literally hated me. He was saying, "You're not a good person – we know that. You take three paces and I will bring you down like you're resisting arrest." It was deliberate. I felt completely violated.'

Finally, the police found what they had been looking for.

'The syringes were sitting on my books on the shelf in the bedroom,' Millar recalled. 'It said Eprex' – an EPO brand name – 'on them. Yeah, I was *really* trying to cover my tracks . . . I'd been sure that they wouldn't find anything but then when they got into the bedroom, I started worrying. I knew there was something on the bookshelves. I started thinking "Oh *fuck* . . ." By then, it was past midnight. They took me to Biarritz prison and left me in a cell on my own for twelve hours.'

But why, given his growing paranoia over phone taps and secret filming, did Millar keep the empty ampoules of EPO on his bookshelves? Was it to prick his guilt every time he came home from a race, to remind him of the innocence that had been lost on his journey from young hopeful to world champion?

Gaumont was sure he had the answer. 'David had kept the syringes even though he knew I had talked to the judge about him and that he was being watched. He told Judge Pallain that it was to never forget that he was a cheat. Knowing David and his sensitivity, I am sure that this is true. I am sure too that, unconsciously, he wanted to be caught – so that it could all stop.'

BURN THIS

July, 2005, central London, on a warm summer evening two days after Lance Armstrong's sixth successive Tour de France victory.

Unshaven, gaunt and with tired eyes, David Millar sits at a pavement table outside a bar in Leicester Square, trying to explain it all away. I am listening to him, but I can't help thinking 'So Gaumont wasn't such a nutter after all, then Dave . . .'

I want to understand, empathise. Fran, his sister, sits beside him, sipping a beer, smoking, occasionally biting her nails. It's only afterwards that I see her presence as a display of solidarity with her vilified brother, the dope cheat. She doesn't say much, just listens and shares the burden of shame and guilt.

David's new life as a self-confessed doper is evidently not easy, however. He tries to play it down. He shrugs, smiles, cracks jokes, still, albeit half-heartedly, the entertainer. At times he laughs a little too hard and long. I sense he is being 'economic' with the truth and still protecting others, while also blaming himself. Later, I learn that his father Gordon had slapped him full in the face over his use of drugs. Now he hangs in limbo, awaiting punishment.

Millar vacantly sips a beer. Across the square, a crowd is building outside a cinema, awaiting the arrival of a clutch of celebs. Passers-by crane their necks. Camera crews set up their equipment. The scene is not unlike the world Millar has now been exiled from, of barriered streets and autograph hunters, of fans waiting patiently, lining up for a snatched glimpse of their heroes.

But David is nobody's hero any more. Because of that night in Biarritz, because of the syringes on the bookshelf, his world has collapsed. Dragged from his cell to the chambers of Judge Pallain, he confessed to doping himself. He was sacked by Cofidis, thrown off the Great British Olympic team for the Athens Games, pursued by the French taxman and sent scurrying back home to England. He is a million miles from that suite in the Bellagio. The British cycling establishment has pilloried him. Millar has been in a lonely place, forced even to sleep on his sister's sofa. 'I've realised who my real friends in cycling are: Baden Cooke, Matt Wilson, Stuart O'Grady, Bobby Julich and Lance. They have all been in touch. That's all, but then a lot of them would probably be scared of calling me . . .'

Lance, says David, was 'lovely to me, he was really good. We talked for ten or fifteen minutes. He was saying, "Keep your head high, it's not the end of the world." He offered help – he said if I needed anything, that I should call him.'

David Millar had once been the great white hope of British cycling, the flag-bearer of a youthful new generation of professionals who had learned the lessons of the post-Festina era.

Looking back though, I realise that prior to his bust, he had always sounded ambivalent. 'Drugs are going to be in sport as long as there's so much money involved,' he told me in 2000. 'You have to make a conscious decision whether to enter into that or not. I've decided I'm not going to enter into that.'

Yet even then, after just two years as a professional, David had sounded unsure. 'I don't know why,' he added. 'It's nothing to do with being a "really decent guy". But it just defeats the purpose for me. I'm a professional, but there are lines that have to be drawn.'

Yet in the end, the decision to dope had been taken easily.

'I went from thinking one hundred per cent that I would never dope to making a decision in ten minutes that I was going to do it. It was an accumulation of things. I wanted to be accepted and to justify my status. Success gave me more power and the ability to control things. But there are so many reasons. It's not black and white. We could talk about it for days, about all the little things, the things in my psychological make-up, the choices I have made.'

The choices . . .?

'I could have been a lot easier on myself by going to live in Nice, but I always wanted to be my own person. I'd train really hard on my own in Biarritz and then hit a slump. There was no "meet the guys at ten in the morning and go and train". If I didn't feel like riding my bike, I didn't ride my bike.'

And then David Millar says this, which, given the wrecking ball through his life his arrest became, is perhaps the saddest thing of all: 'I could have had a good career without doping – it is possible.'

When he finally appeared in court, in late 2006, David Millar stuck to his original statement. He repeated what he'd told me, that doping came through facing up to his 'responsibilities', and thinking that he owed something to his team and sponsor.

'I was getting paid a lot of money to guarantee my results. The management made it clear that I had a lot of responsibilities. But the first time I doped it had nothing to do with money. I didn't even understand my contract very well at the time. I didn't even know that I could have had a one hundred per cent increase in my salary with twenty more UCI points. I blame myself – I assume responsibility for what I have done. But I feel let down and taken advantage of, because Cofidis took a lot of liberties. They screwed up. They can remember how I arrived at the team, nineteen years old. I was so naive, so naive. It was my dream and I didn't realise how good I was. They had nothing for me.'

Cofidis, he says, must have known that he was flirting with disaster, yet they did not intervene. 'They're not stupid,' says David, as he signals to the waiter for another beer. 'They were running a professional cycling team.'

Did doping become a safety net to ensure results when you were short of training or out of form?

'No – this is the paradox. When you boost your performance artificially you become ten times more serious than you have ever been. You don't screw up. You say, "This is no longer sport – this is my job." The moment you dope, you become ten times more professional.'

THE CLEAN MACHINE

Julian Clark sits in a gastropub in Kent, fiddling with his club sandwich. There is an uncharacteristic pause. Normally Julian talks non-stop, but today, he is choosing his words carefully. Memories of his three years managing the Linda McCartney Cycling Team are flooding back.

Most of them are not good.

Clark has an extraordinary story to tell. Almost single-handedly, he converted a weekend shopping trip to Sainsbury's into a groundbreaking opportunity in international sports sponsorship. His whimsical idea of creating a British cycling team that could race the Tour de France became a reality. Julian drove the Linda McCartney cycling team to the brink of European success – and then steered his runaway train into a precipice.

Julian once sent me a draft for a book called *Debt, Drugs and Eating Meat*, which is a blunt but accurate summary of his journey from infatuated cycling fan to bankruptcy and breakdown. He has always been a seat-of-the-pants character. He finished racing in motocross in 1990, after a bad crash left him with a blood clot on the brain. He was only twenty-five. After a year's recovery, he started racing in triathlons. 'I enjoyed the bike-racing part the most,' he recalls. 'Various people told me that I was strong on the bike and that I should do some road racing.'

He adjusted well to serious competition. 'I was a fourth-category amateur but I rode a race called the Les England Memorial down in Bletchingley and Chris Lillywhite, John Tanner – all the relevant elite riders in Britain – were there. I'd already had a win in a second-cat race, but that day I got into a breakaway with Lillywhite and the others and was still there at the end, before I blew up – big time.'

But Clark had earned their respect and he and Lillywhite became friends. 'They all came and talked to me afterwards and said I was strong, so I started training with Chris, because we lived locally to each other. I was completely smitten with the sport, overwhelmed. I thought it was fantastic. I'd come from pro racing in motocross to cycling and I wanted to be a pro bike rider.'

During his time in motocross, Clark had taken managerial roles and proved adept at attracting sponsors. Now, as an established rider on the parochial British racing scene, he wanted to do the same in cycling.

'In March 1998, Tracey and I were wandering around Sainsbury's in Cobham. I was just looking through the frozen foods, saw Linda McCartney's brand and realised what they were about. I thought her brand and cycling would be a great match. So Tracey and I sat up until whatever time it was that night, putting a proposal together for the sponsorship of a cycling team and sent it off.'

Incredibly, they struck gold. 'Less than two weeks later we met with Paul McCartney and the deal for 1998 was done.'

Fuelled by his good fortune, Clark didn't hang about: he tracked down a group of British professionals who were racing abroad, met them at a café in Cobham, and promised them a job. Three weeks later, he had a team car from Rover, six riders (including himself in the role of player/manager), a clothing sponsor and a schedule of racing, which included some brief European sorties.

'We'd got back from the Tour of Slovenia, only our fourth race, and were racing in Gloucester. But we got a call that night saying that Linda had died.'

Despite Linda McCartney's death, the sponsorship deal remained intact. 'We were told that Paul wanted the team to carry on as Linda's legacy. She had always been very hands-on

– there were pictures of us all with her published in the *Sun* – she was very taken with cycling. She said to me, "I want to see this team in the Tour de France."'

Clark says that although some of the momentum was lost with Linda McCartney's death, the team's ambitions grew. Further sponsors came on board in 1999, as did a new *directeur sportif*, Sean Yates. Motorola, keen to promote the advantages to families of their communication equipment, was one new sponsor.

Clark and Yates put together a new squad of fourteen riders. Julian became general manager, running the team full-time, as the riders competed in a mixture of Premier Calendar races in Britain and a few B-list races abroad. Slowly but surely, it was all coming together.

Yates, a stage winner in the Tour de France and one of the most highly regarded British professionals, had been nudging towards his fortieth birthday when he came out of retirement to race in the Tour of Britain for Clark and the team. 'He did a good job for us,' Clark recalls, 'and brought us a lot of publicity.'

I knew Yates well. He was one of the first riders I interviewed. He could be monosyllabic and blunt, but we got on well enough and became friendly. For the final phase of his career I ghosted a Yates column. When he retired, he invited me to his house on the edge of Ashdown Forest for dinner, opening a choice bottle of wine as we talked across the dining table. His knowledge of the races and riders was detailed and analytical, his view of racing pragmatic and unromantic. When that seam of conversation ran dry we would talk about gardening, his other great passion.

Occasionally he would be more animated. In the uncertain atmosphere that followed the Festina Affair, relations between us became more awkward. For one of the columns, I asked him for his perspective on doping. After what had happened, would he want his kids to go into bike racing? I asked.

Yates quickly grew exasperated. 'I'm sick of this shit,' he blurted. 'We're all just trying to do our jobs.'

By British standards, Yates was a high achiever, with veteran status in the European peloton, a reputation for brutal self-criticism and some good connections. In the final few years of his career, he had ridden for the Motorola team alongside a youthful Lance Armstrong. On the European circuit, they were often room-mates. Yates had shown the young Texan the ropes, staved off his bouts of homesickness, calmed him down when he got hot-headed and developed his tactical awareness.

Little by little, Yates rounded the rough edges off the redneck, giving him a new understanding of European etiquette. They became so close that Lance even came to stay at Yates' house in Forest Row, training with the Englishman back and forth on the climbs through Ashdown Forest.

With Yates on board, it all seemed to be coming together. Julian began dreaming of European success.

'The whole ethos was that we were the "Clean Machine". There were the vegetarian foods, we were eco-friendly – these guys can win on a lettuce, that kind of thing. McCartney had even written a song, "Clean Machine", for our website.'

Only a handful of British professionals have proved capable of racing in Europe. Some of them, like Yates, stayed the course and lasted a decade or so, while others struggled to learn the language, failed to get results and finally returned home.

Matt Stephens was a highly talented British pro, a former national champion, capable of far more than simply eking out a living on the stuttering British circuit, something he combined with his job as a customer services manager for Marks & Spencer in Chester. Seven years after the demise of his European career, and now a police officer, when I ask him if he knew of any professional riders who were doping, he says, 'I think people who have doped – people who haven't doped – will still say to you that they don't want to make any comment, not because they want the sport to continue the way it is, but because people are frightened of saying anything and getting their livelihood taken away from them.'

At thirty-eight, he still loves cycling and races regularly on the British circuit. He manages to balance work, family and training, squeezing in about ten hours' training a week.

Like others before him, he had always dreamed of racing in Europe, but thought the chance had passed him by. So when, in 1999, he was made an offer by the Linda McCartney team, it didn't take long to make a decision.

'I'd almost given up when the McCartneys hired me, because I was nearly thirty. I was at peak form and my natural strength was at its highest. I was pretty much the number one on the UK circuit.'

Stephens had been riding for a Harrods-sponsored team until the middle of 1999. 'There was a mutual respect between Sean Yates and myself and I'd had contact with him and Julian. The McCartney guys were taking it to another level and they offered me a rolling contract to the end of the season.'

Stephens did well enough to be offered a 'good deal' for 2000. 'It was good enough to pack in my day job. It was something I'd always wanted to do and something that I knew probably wouldn't come around again.'

He was paid an initial salary of £20,000, plus occasional bonuses. 'To be honest, that was what a lot of the guys on the team were on at that time. I had no illusions, but I couldn't have accepted anything less than that. I was hopeful of developing it and staying pro for five or six years, building up to something quite reasonable. With a sponsor like McCartney and people like Sean on board, I was pretty certain it would continue. It looked like a good proposition.'

The highpoint of Stephens' year with the McCartneys came at the 2000 Giro d'Italia. 'It was the peak of my career really. I was on the start ramp for the prologue among all the guys I'd admired growing up. It was no mean feat for a British rider.

I was so chuffed, being there with Marco Pantani and the others.'

The fact that the day before the prologue, Stephens, like all the riders in the Giro field, had been invited to an audience with the Pope, illustrates the importance of cycling to Italian life. 'Eddy Merckx was there as well. I'm not a religious person, but that in itself, going to the Vatican, was quite awe-inspiring.'

Stephens remembers that during that Giro there was a great team spirit among the McCartneys. 'We had a good laugh, although I was disappointed because I crashed early and was basically getting through each day.'

In the end, despite his best efforts, he was forced to quit the race in the final week, almost within sight of the race finish in Milan. 'I cried,' he recalls. 'To get that far, given the condition that I was in, was still fantastic.'

Yet it was on that Giro that Stephens realised the extent of cycling's dark side.

'You are aware of what's going on. It is an eye-opener. But Britain is an island – we've got a different culture. For example, British Cycling has this academy – you can ride clean with the academy but end up abroad where they've got a completely different ethic. I know that it's just so corrupt.'

Even now? I ask. 'There're guys now who are preaching who I know have been some of the worst abusers of drugs. EPO use was pretty rife – everybody knows that. We were quite rigorously tested by the "vampires". [The Giro] was edgy, because you knew that certain individuals were doing it, that hotels were raided by the police. It had got to the stage where you knew you could end up inside. It was quite frightening, but it was just glossed over by the glamour of the sport.'

Stephens admits that he was tempted to dope, but he didn't. 'It's there, it's available if you want to go down that route. People have got to make decisions, but the temptation was there because you knew how much difference it could make. I'd worn the British champion's jersey clean and I thought "Why can't I continue like that?" But then you go to Italy and it's like, *shiiit* – it's just another level entirely. Climbing the mountains you think "This is impossible – what's going on?" There's a big gap in performance if you're not taking anything. And you could still technically take EPO at that time, as long as you were sensible with your levels.'

Stephens has been depressed by the doping scandals of recent years. He is in favour of the introduction of DNA testing as a means of establishing blood profiles. Others are not convinced. Some leading riders are against DNA testing on principle – it's an invasion of privacy, they say, we're not common criminals. But that reticence clearly rankles.

'Why the hell shouldn't riders give a DNA sample? As a police officer I had to give a DNA sample otherwise they wouldn't let me have the job. You can say that it's an infringement of human rights, but if you have got nothing to hide and you love your sport – and you're not doing the gear – then what's the problem?'

In the end, Stephens' own European dream was short-lived. The unravelling of the Linda McCartney team in January 2001, when Julian Clark's promises of continuing sponsorship came to nothing, was, he says, 'awful'.

Until Clark's last stand, Stephens had believed he'd agreed a contract with the team for 2001. 'I felt like I'd been punched in the stomach. I had a mortgage to pay and no job. I had to sign on.

'Julian was a very chatty guy and I got on with him well. I considered him a friend and I think he had the best intentions. He had the patter and a hell of a lot of drive. His intention was to realise a dream. At the end of the day, we rode a Grand Tour and we rode some brilliant races, but we didn't know the truth about the finances. He did very well in shielding us from that.

'I just wish he'd have handled it differently. What he should have done was told us that he couldn't guarantee a team for the next year and that we could go out and look for other teams to ride for. But I think he had dug such a hole that he couldn't get out of it.

'I know he had initial talks with Jaguar and Jacob's Creek . . . but on the back of that, he basically bankrolled the team with loans in lieu of sponsorship money that was never going to turn up.

'The primary thing was the name McCartney – we thought it was invincible. But it wasn't.'

There were thirty-five to forty full- and part-time jobs lost in the debacle, with Julian Clark seen as the villain of the piece.

'The worst part was that I'd spoken with Dave Millar that summer at the National Championships and he'd asked me if I'd like to ride for Cofidis the following year. I'd said, "Yeah, I'd love to," but also that I believed in the way the McCartney team was going and was hoping to build it up for the next year. So I turned down a ride with Dave . . . But on the other hand,' says Matt Stephens, 'look what happened to Cofidis and Dave – maybe that was fate intervening.'

THE END OF THE AFFAIR

As the 2000 season loomed, Clark was torn between remaining a big fish in a small pond, by developing the team as a UK and USA squad, or trying his luck in Europe, where risks were higher, but rewards far greater. Once Julian had taken the plunge and opted for Europe, he moved the team to the south of France, near Toulouse. The stakes had got higher. Julian and his team were now committed to winning at the elite level.

Toulouse, with an international airport and a good motorway network, was an ideal location. 'It was far easier to get back and forth from races in Europe. From England, with a limited budget, you can't do it.'

Clark moved his wife, Tracey, and their two kids out to France and set up an office and a *service course*, or team warehouse, for equipment and spare parts. The team's budget had increased by only £150,000, but Clark remained optimistic of further sponsorship.

'There was an ongoing plan for Heinz to come on board. McVitie's had the licence to sell and distribute Linda McCartney foods, but they were only sold in the UK. For the Linda brand to be sold worldwide, Heinz planned to buy the frozen-food division of McVitie's, including Linda McCartney foods. It was supposed to be done before the 2000 season and they were going to come in to enable us to go to the next level. But this dragged on and on. Meantime, I'd gone to Toulouse, set up there, was signing riders and planning to develop the team.' To keep things going until the

Heinz–McVitie's deal came through, and to ensure the Tour de France dream remained alive, Clark set up an overdraft to cover the shortfall.

Half a dozen or so more experienced riders came on board for the 2000 season. These included Max Sciandri, the Anglo-Italian rider and Olympic medallist, who now works for British Cycling, Swiss Pascal Richard, a veteran stage-race rider and winner of the Olympic road race at the Atlanta Games, Norwegian Bjornar Vestol, Italian Maurizio De Pasquale and Tayeb Braikia from Denmark.

The 2000 Giro d'Italia proved to be a deep-end experience for Julian Clark. The pressure on him to land more sponsorship was intense and his balancing act grew more precarious by the day. 'My overdraft was up to here,' he says, raising his hand above his head. 'I was still paying the riders out of my Lloyds bank account. I was sitting in the back of the team car on the phone to the bank every day. It was horrendous.'

Unexpectedly, the team won a stage in the Giro through David McKenzie, and then took second place in the following day's stage. That made Clark increasingly convinced that, surely, Heinz would come on board. 'But,' Julian says, with some understatement, 'I think maybe I was being over-optimistic.'

Working alongside Clark at the Giro was assistant *directeur* Chris Lillywhite. Both men were taken aback by the doping practices they encountered at that year's race. 'I was like, "This is how it is – this is what real cycling is," said Lillywhite. "This is what's behind the real sport." It becomes the normal thing to do, rather than the extraordinary thing to do.'

Lillywhite has very little involvement in professional cycling these days. He works in London as a plumber and he's busy on jobs most of the week. On his days off he heads off to Stamford Bridge to watch Chelsea. He says he's out of touch with cycling, that he was only ever a 'small-time' pro, but as a former Milk Race winner and one of the outstanding riders of his generation, his name still resonates with British cycling fans.

'I was a small-time rider based in the UK,' he remembers. 'The drugs thing was there but it wasn't prolific when I was a rider. In the 1980s there was maybe a little bit of amphetamine going around. I would say it was quite innocent compared to how things are now.

'From being a small-time rider on small teams, and then being catapulted into European cycling, did open my eyes to the fact that to get on and compete with the best, you had to be "preparing" yourself. They call it "the programme" – whether that's taking illegal substances is down to how you interpret it. But it opened my eyes to how involved the medical side was.

'I'd played at racing for ten years in the UK, but it was easy street. You know, you ride around for an hour in a city centre, pick up your money – but then you go to Europe and see guys busting their balls, doing all sorts of stuff to their body and quite often, not even making as much money as we were in the UK. They wanted to climb the ladder, to get to the top.

'I never took any drugs during my career. As far as my sporting career goes, I never felt I needed to, because I wasn't at that level.

'But,' he says, 'I'd do it now, one hundred per cent. Because looking back at my career, I feel like I underachieved and I feel like I could have done a little bit better, I could have got a European contract.

'I didn't have the hunger to do it – I wasn't willing to do what it took. I think I could have achieved a lot more. If that had involved some sort of medical programme, then, looking back, I would have done it.'

The only time I ever travelled with the Linda McCartney team on a European race day turned into a very strange day indeed. Julian arranged a seat in the number one team car driven by

Sean Yates at the Belgian Classic, Ghent-Wevelgem. At the first feed zone of the race, I hopped into the passenger seat alongside Sean when he pulled over to pick up more food and drink from the team *soigneurs*.

Yates flung the car back into the race convoy and I quickly realised that things weren't going well. Spencer Smith, the former world triathlon champion, who was hoping to break into road racing, had been the first to quit, and Max Sciandri, supposedly the team's Classics specialist, was having an off day.

Things got worse. Sciandri was left behind by the front group of riders and found himself racing in no-man's-land. At one point he was overtaken by a muscular one-legged rider in Cofidis kit, a moment that did little for Max's already fragile ego. Later, David Millar told me that his Cofidis team also sponsored a high-achieving, amputee paralympian, who often snuck onto the back of race convoys to test himself against the pros.

Race radio wasn't working well either. Madonna occasionally crackled across the short-wave announcements as the signal came and went, filling the team car with doodling beats as we strained for news of what was happening at the front of the race. When the race radio's signal finally came back, we found out that Erik Zabel, then leader of the Telekom team, had crashed − after an encounter with a rogue pony.

Sciandri meanwhile rode on, but his mood was sombre. Off the pace, off the back, out of contention − Sciandri's failure spoke volumes about the team's true place in cycling's pecking order. Finally, after he'd dropped further behind, Yates pulled alongside his team leader once more.

'Is that it?' he bellowed bluntly at Sciandri. Max braked and slowed to a halt, clipping his feet out of the pedals in one motion. He climbed into the team car with barely a word. I was demoted to the back seat. Max sat beside Sean, his defences up, adopting the monosyllabic sulk that characterised other disappointing moments in his career. We drove on to the finish, passing US

Postal's Frankie Andreu, Yates' old Motorola teammate, further along the road. Yates slowed the car, wound down a window and called out a greeting. The American looked across with weary eyes.

'Oh – hi Sean,' responded Andreu, disinterestedly, as he pedalled on towards the finish.

Julian Clark's grand design finally collapsed in January 2001. Crippled by lack of sponsorship, the Linda McCartney team fell apart at its pre-season get-together. The financial insecurities that Julian had battled to stave off came home to roost. There was no deal with Heinz. All the broken promises and missed payments turned team personnel against him. Julian went to ground. In the fallout, he took most of the blame, his defence further undermined by his absence, he says through illness, from the final painful meetings in a hotel in Surrey.

Clark had been undone by his own reckless ambition and by some ill-conceived strategies. The straw that broke the camel's back may have been his decision to bring retired former Festina rider, Neil Stephens, to the team as a sports director alongside Yates.

Stephens had always maintained his innocence of any wrongdoing, but the Australian's connections to the Festina Affair in 1998 made his appointment foolhardy. After all the fuss, Stephens only really worked for the McCartneys on one race – the 2001 Tour Down Under. More importantly for Clark's bank balance and for the future of his team, the negative publicity, both in Britain and Australia, over somebody from *that team* mentoring young riders, appeared to give potential sponsor Jacob's Creek cold feet.

Not that the winemaker was expected to provide hard cash. As 2001 began, the Heinz deal, with a budget of £1.7 million, was still supposedly about to drop into place, so Julian optimistically offered Jacob's Creek the chance to sponsor the team – free of charge. 'I said, "We'll show you what we can

97

do, with a view to 2002."' He was also talking to Jaguar and, taking a chance, decided to order team clothing with both brands prominently displayed. All of it turned out to be wishful thinking.

'I was driving around the *péripherique* in Toulouse with Tracey, and I got a call from the marketing director at Heinz in the States. "Me and the guys have had a meeting and we're not going to go ahead with the team."' Julian exploded. 'I'd always shown this guy a lot of respect and brown-nosed a bit, but I just said, "What the *fuck* do you mean?! What am I supposed to do now?" And he said, "I suggest you take this up with Sir Paul . . ."'

In the end, the stress of it all overwhelmed Julian. At the time, it was reported that he had suffered a heart attack, but he says this was not the case. Instead, his mind and body fried by the nervous exhaustion of the previous few months, he became a recluse. He was widely blamed by the Linda McCartney riders and staff, vilified as a chancer and con man in the British cycling press and publicly criticised by both Sean Yates and Neil Stephens. Some of it, he acknowledges, was deserved, but nonetheless all of it hurt. His overdraft, he claims, stood at £180,000 when the team folded. In a matter of weeks, he was declared bankrupt.

In the aftermath, Julian was depressed, but he was angry too. He still hadn't given up, even if, in his desperation, the situation now became as comic as it was tragic. 'I thought, well, what if I could come up with a replacement sponsor to support the British riders and me?'

After flying the flag for vegetarianism, his first port of call was, quite naturally, British Meat. Julian must have thought his luck was in when his pitch was well received by the marketing director, Alan Lamb, but events conspired against him. 'Then came the foot and mouth outbreak,' he recalls, 'and that was that.'

It could have been so different. Maybe the team could have carried on racing at home, as a low-key British-based operation.

'I could have stayed a big fish in a small pond and earned a fair amount of money out of it,' he reasons.

But he doesn't really believe that any major sponsor would have supported a UK-based team. 'How can you ever take a sponsor to a British race?' he asks. 'You can't – not one race. There's nobody there. And anyone who is there, is out of the ark.'

Julian maintains that if Jacob's Creek had taken the team on, if Heinz had committed, and if Neil Stephens had been able to escape the ghosts of his past, then maybe the Linda McCartney team would still be going. 'I really wanted the team to succeed. We knew that there was a short window of publicity because of the McCartney name and that was only going to last a little while before we were going to need results. It became very quickly apparent that there was *no chance* of getting results in Europe, unless they were doing what the others were doing. No question . . .'

You mean doping? I say.

Julian nods.

Julian Clark still loves cycling. He spent most of the summer of 2006 racing in the Surrey League series. He ended up winning his age group – 'clean, of course,' he points out.

The simplicity and innocence of the British club scene appeals to him. 'It's nice. I'll ride out to local races from home, have a chat in the changing rooms, race hard all day. And they're all clean.'

Julian couldn't quite believe, after all the years ducking and diving, trying to get into the Tour de France, that the Tour de France came to him; the first road stage of the 2007 Tour, which started in central London, passed his front door in Kent. Unsurprisingly, the irony tickled him. He fired up his barbecue, invited some friends over and watched the race go past.

And after the Tour had gone, Julian gathered up the empties, packed away the charcoal, went back indoors and got on with his life.

THE ENTOURAGE

My phone beeps. Perhaps not for the first time in his life, Alastair Campbell is feeling rather pleased with himself.

'Meeting Lance was great. If there's anything I can ever do, let me know,' he texted. I gazed out of the window at the north London drizzle and pondered the prospect of Tony Blair's legendary spin doctor becoming my own personal fixer. No letters ever, ever again from the Inland Revenue? A pledge to desist from his 'Evening With . . .' tours around Britain? Most importantly of all, a promise to steer clear of any future British Lions tours?

In the spring of 2004, *The Times* sports desk called asking if I could finesse an introduction to Lance Armstrong on behalf of Campbell. After exiting Number 10 in wake of the 'dodgy dossier' farrago that had polarised opinion on the wisdom of the war in Iraq, Campbell had returned to journalism. He was compiling a list of his greatest athletes. Armstrong was among them.

By the time Lance had won his fifth Tour in 2003, with a display of tenacity and rage that shocked even those who knew him well, he had become a people's hero. His charitable deeds, his books – the first of which, *It's Not About the Bike*, had become a global bestseller – had given him a profile which transcended his sport. He was somebody in Hollywood, a regular on Letterman and Leno – able to count Bono, George Bush, Sandra Bullock, Matthew McConaughey, Robin Williams and Sheryl Crow among his best friends.

It's Not About the Bike is a powerfully told story, expertly turned by ghostwriter Sally Jenkins. It develops the notion of

Lance as an avenging angel – and the idea that somehow each Tour win further righted the wrongs and slights committed against the sick and helpless. This had real resonance in the United States, particularly in the post-9/11 era and the build-up to the invasion of Iraq, when America grew more isolated from the rest of the world. When Lance spoke of overcoming cancer and fighting against the odds to audiences at fundraising events, many listening would be moved to tears.

By this time Lance had transcended his sport to become a highly paid motivational guru in a sharp suit. The baseball-cap-wearing, sweatshirted, bullshit-free redneck that I had first met in Leeds was now unrecognisable. On his last couple of Tours, I had struggled to convince myself that it was *actually him* out there in Lycra, pedalling and jostling, cursing and spitting, getting sweaty and tired, sore-arsed and fly-spattered. Didn't he have somebody else to do this stuff? I'd take a stroll down to the team bus at the start village in the mornings, just to check it was really him. And yes – I can confirm that it genuinely was Lance Armstrong who rode all of those seven triumphant Tours.

The US Postal team bus was the hub of Lancemania. Bodyguards, camera crews, fans and groupies milled around. If you were lucky you might get a word with Sheryl or Robin. There was one band of stateside fans, 'The Cutters', who hung out by the bus, whooping things up every morning with '*Yewdamaaan!*'-style hollering. 'The Cutters' were modelled on the wrong-side-of-the-tracks kids in the movie *Breaking Away*. The first year they showed up on the Tour, I ran into them late one night in a pizzeria in the Pyrenees, sunburnt, exhausted and scraping together enough loose change to pay the bill. Within a couple of years they were transformed into official Lance cheerleaders, with endorsement contracts of their own.

It's Not About the Bike won the William Hill Sports Book of the Year award in Britain and had become something of a self-help bible. It had an enormous impact, perhaps even a greater impact than his Tour wins. Around the dinner table, people would say that they didn't really like cycling, but they 'loved Lance's amazing book'.

Armstrong and his agent, Bill Stapleton, had realised their dream. In the five years since making his comeback, Lance had become an icon. Stapleton told me after Lance's second Tour win that the 'brand was more mature'. By 2004, it was more than mature – it was global.

It was more than a brand to those who were close to Armstrong: it was a gravy train. The longer he maintained his position at the top of the sport, the richer they all became. And the more global the Lance brand became, the more distant he grew. My own relationship with him was virtually non-existent by this time, partly because direct contact with him was blocked by The Entourage, partly because there was no 'exclusive' time to be had any more, and partly because he had taken umbrage at my criticism of his ongoing relationship with Michele Ferrari. 'I can choose who I talk to and I chose not to talk to him,' Lance told Stapleton in an email that his agent then forwarded to me. It ended: 'I actually think he's an OK guy.' But that didn't tally with other accounts. The garrulous, sometimes indiscreet, Texan journalist, Suzanne Halliburton had revealed that Lance had described me to her as 'a snake with arms'.

When I heard that, I was, as they say, pretty pissed, but even then it made me smile and think of him with a flicker of grudging affection. The insult carried a characteristic touch of paranoia as if I had somehow betrayed him, slithering into his inner circle, before turning it to my advantage. The 'snake with arms' – maybe it was a mythical backwoods creature from the Texas Hill Country, maybe it was the ultimate Austin insult. Maybe it was a bumper sticker – 'Don't Mess With The Snake With Arms.'

I'm not really sure where Lance and I parted company. It was a gradual freezing out, but even at the end of the 1999 Tour, it was clear that things were changing. As the race headed for Paris, I had called him. We chatted about his victory as he sat in the back of a team car wending its way down the hairpins from Alpe d'Huez to Bourg d'Oisans. We finished the conversation remembering how frail he had been during the mid-chemo visit to the house on Lake Austin.

'I feel like I made a part of the journey with you,' I said.

'That's right,' he responded, 'you did.'

When I tried to call him a few weeks later, his cellphone was unattainable. I called the office in Austin. Access was denied. I'd have to talk to Stapleton and book a time to speak to Lance. They weren't giving out his number to anybody – *not anybody*. Now it was my turn to be paranoid: with the big American networks and *Sports Illustrated* beating a path to his door, I wondered if I had served my purpose.

The distance between us grew.

It became a divide during the 2001 Tour, when Armstrong and David Walsh of the *Sunday Times* went head to head in an electrifying press conference at the Palais des Congrès in Pau over the Texan's relationship with Michele Ferrari. The Italian was facing a trial in Italy on doping charges. Walsh, following a series of vitriolic articles that had pursued Armstrong over his credibility, scented blood. Almost a decade earlier, the pair had struck up a rapport when Walsh had met the American and been impressed, like me, by his brazen charm and youthful directness.

But Armstrong, vintage 2001, was more complex.

On the road his mastery was complete; off the road he sometimes needed a little help from his friends in the press. For most of the Tour, he had deflected the endless questions over his contacts with Ferrari, which climaxed in the head to head with Walsh in Pau, using subtle sledging towards his rivals, and vague accusations of unprofessionalism.

Prior to the final Tour time trial in 2001, he was scathing about Jan Ullrich's level of pre-Tour preparation. 'Where was Ullrich when I was here in April, in the pissing rain, riding the time-trial course?'

But then the Armstrong-Ferrari–Bruyneel combination always

went to extraordinary lengths to defend their supremacy. Nothing was left to chance. Forget the allegations of doping (always fiercely denied, and backed up by countless negative dope tests): there were other incidents that summed up their collective attitude towards the spirit of fair play.

Armstrong understood that Ferrari was notoriously indiscreet. As the mystery about him grew, the tales about him achieved the status of urban myths. He was once supposedly spotted racing in a triathlon in Lavarone, wearing a fake race number, illegally 'pacing' his daughter, Sara, while she competed for the Italian national team.

Despite his unassuming appearance, Ferrari's ego demanded recognition. Among his most famous gaffes, was his own revelation that he would 'talk' Armstrong through the Tour, simply by watching the race on TV. 'Lance calls me from his bike,' Ferrari told Danish newspaper *Ekstra Bladet*.

During the Alpine stages of the 2000 Tour, as Marco Pantani did his damnedest to dethrone the champion, Ferrari advised the American via a link from Bruyneel's mobile phone to Armstrong's in-race radio earpiece. When Pantani attacked, Ferrari, watching in front of his TV screen at home in Italy, told Armstrong to remain calm and not to waste energy, because he believed that the Italian had overreached himself. And Ferrari was proved right.

'Obviously it wasn't good to let Pantani go,' recalled Armstrong. 'But how fast was he really going? How long could he sustain that? And Ferrari would know the answer to that, because he is above all a mathematician. A brilliant mathematician with a ton of experience.'

This was the Tour de France by remote control.

If Greg LeMond's interpretation was that the Italian was a 'crazed scientist', Armstrong preferred to call Ferrari 'misunderstood'.

He described Ferrari as 'very, very smart', but also acknowledged that he was prone to painful gaffes. Ferrari, Lance said, had 'made some incredibly bad mistakes in terms of press and interviews, and the way he reacted to certain questions. I've known him for a long time and . . . we've known him to be fair and honest and correct and ethical, so we cannot punish the guy, because that's the person we see.'

The Italian case against Ferrari over doping offences was, Armstrong said, trumped up. 'It wouldn't make it through the first five minutes in a court in the United States of America, where you have ethics and you have codes, and you have laws and you have judges that are unbiased . . . Ferrari's not getting a fair shake.'

Lance later used similar language when, in 2005, *L'Equipe* published allegations – which Lance fiercely denied – that EPO had been present in his urine samples during the 1999 Tour. After this, would he ever return to France? he was asked: 'No way. I wouldn't get a fair shake in France on the roadside, in the doping controls, or in the lab.' Yet Armstrong had praised the same French anti-doping laboratory, at Châtenay-Malabry in Paris, in 2004 and described it as having 'an excellent reputation'.

In Pau on that July afternoon in 2001, Walsh and Armstrong linked their fates, like a latter day Captain Ahab and Moby Dick. The press conference had begun amiably enough, an American journalist asking Lance about chateaux and wine, the German media asking him for an assessment of Jan Ullrich. Then Armstrong looked up to see that Walsh was the next questioner.

'Glad you could make it, David,' growled Lance.

It was an extraordinary encounter, Walsh on the offensive, Lance maintaining his cool, their positions entrenched by mutual loathing. The Irishman appeared willing to stake his reputation on his ability to topple the icon, to force him into submission. But Armstrong was too tough to fold in front of us all and gladly locked horns with him.

He defended the Italian: 'I've never denied the relationship. I believe Dr Ferrari's an honest man. Until somebody's proven guilty, then I see them as innocent. If there's a conviction then we will re-evaluate the relationship.'

In response, Walsh raged at Armstrong, like a demented Catholic priest – '*Yew preeesent yerself as the cleaaanest of the cleaaan!*' he bellowed in his high brogue – but the Texan didn't buckle. The confrontation was a tie. When it was over, Lance strode out into the afternoon sunshine, Stapleton and The Entourage – PR men, brand managers, personal assistants, bodyguards and sunglasses reps – hot on his heels. He stepped into a US Postal Service team car, no doubt turning the air blue as he was sped away. After that, every Armstrong press conference was strictly controlled.

Nonetheless, Walsh's tirade had gained him some support. Allied to Ferrari's long-standing ambivalence over doping, Armstrong's admissions of regular contacts with the Italian and his refusal to distance himself from him during the doping trial all provoked debate.

Lance had constantly played down the Ferrari connection, yet seemed prepared to risk his image over the relationship. Was Walsh a fantasist? Was Greg LeMond simply as bitter as some said?

And even then, even if they were both as wrong as The Entourage insisted they were, why wouldn't Lance and Stapleton, now so focussed on the global appeal of the Armstrong brand, ditch Ferrari until the court case was over? Why was Lance so fiercely loyal to him?

I watched the camera crews film Armstrong's departure, turned back to see Walsh holding court in a huddle of journalists with notebooks, and realised that I would soon have to choose sides.

Alastair Campbell and Lance Armstrong had some similarities. Both had undergone a rebirth of sorts. An evangelical chord had been struck between them; Campbell, once a hard-drinking, stressed-out hack but now a born-again athlete, had, like so many, been smitten with the recovered, near-evangelical cancer victim and had seen a parallel in his own battle for redemption and understanding.

There was another strand of empathy between them. Both believed themselves to be misunderstood and misrepresented.

They loathed journalists and the mainstream media, particularly when they strayed off message. As Campbell wrote, a little pompously, in his *Times* piece: 'Armstrong was attracted to meeting someone who feels even more deeply about the press and its misrepresentations than he does.'

It was ironic, then, given that Campbell was writing for *The Times*, that Armstrong's media nemesis was Walsh, chief sports writer on the *Sunday Times*.

I pondered on whether it was legitimate to use Campbell's interest in Armstrong to my own advantage. But, ostracised by The Entourage, I didn't ponder for long. So I called him.

I told Campbell about Lance's professionalism, his frightening focus, about how he'd taken cycling to a whole new level of wealth and prestige. With a lot of British media outlets now shunned by Armstrong in the aftermath of the Walsh confrontation, I told him that, yes, I was sure Lance would love to meet Tony Blair's former right-hand man, but that things with the British media were delicately poised.

But I also knew that Lance, friend and Texan neighbour to 'Dubya', would respond positively to an invitation from somebody so close to Blair. This way he would have both sides of the transatlantic alliance covered – an 'in' with both the White House and Number 10.

Stapleton soon warmed to Campbell's interest in Lance. Earlier when I'd embarked on a charm offensive it had taken days to get a reply. Not this time. A few hours later Armstrong's agent responded: 'Lance would be happy to do this.'

Campbell and Armstrong finally got together in Lance's apartment in Girona in north-east Spain. He had moved there with Kristin and the kids after the atmosphere towards him in France, both from the media and the public, had become overwhelmingly hostile. But now his wife and three children were long gone, and when Campbell turned up, Sheryl Crow was at

Armstrong's side. I had negotiated access for a photographer, a rare privilege, but *The Times* ran only a couple of images. In contrast, *procycling* published almost a dozen. Lance, a confirmed atheist, posed a little eerily in front of the chapel he'd created for his Catholic ex-wife. This was the king in his castle.

'Losing and dying,' he told Campbell at one point. 'It's the same thing.'

The pictures showed Campbell and Crow sipping coffee and Lance and Alastair pottering in his bike workshop. Lance, prompted by Sheryl, ribbed Campbell about those weapons of mass destruction. Campbell defended himself and Blair. Lance, Sheryl and Alastair all agreed that President Bush was actually quite a bright guy and not at all like his public image.

Campbell did pause on Armstrong's fight to clear his name against the rumours of doping, and Lance trotted out the usual defences. He was the most tested athlete on the planet and he'd never tested positive. It was a French conspiracy, he said, a witch-hunt. The French media were anti-American, even more so in the aftermath of the Iraq war. They were bitter after losing the Tour for so many years and were now so cynical that they couldn't believe his story. Campbell wrote: 'I'm not bad at reading people and either he's a good liar or telling the truth.'

It made for an intriguing read, even if it had the tone of a press release in parts. It was unquestioning, and accepting of the Armstrong legend, of the tenets of hard work, commitment and desire. Lance even pulled out some new bumper stickers: 'Go hard or go home,' he told Campbell, when asked for any tips for young athletes.

'*Don't Mess With Texas, Go Hard or Go Home, Ride Like Ya Stole Something, Live Strong . . .*'

The more interviews Lance gave, the more of these inanities he trotted out. On a slow afternoon, we would sit around in the *procycling* office coming up with clichés in the style of Lance. Travel writer, raconteur and cycling anorak, Tim Moore, who spent some long hours with me in the Tour car one year, was annoyingly good at the daytime TV self-help platitudes that Armstrong often resorted to.

'*Hey — I climbed a mountain and when I got to the top, I met a guy I liked. And you know what? That guy was me!*' Tim intoned in a flat, bored drawl as we motored onwards through the Alps.

We weren't alone; in response to the epidemic of 'Livestrong' wristbands covering the planet, a website selling 'Livewrong' wristbands, T-shirts and baseball caps soon popped up. As ever, Lance demanded a reaction; he didn't leave people indifferent to him.

Campbell and I talked again as that year's Tour ended in Paris. Could I arrange accreditation for him for the final stage? He wanted to write a piece on Lance's historic win and was hopeful he'd be able to have a chat with The Great Man too. Late at night on the Tour's final Saturday, as we drove north towards Paris, my phone flashed in the darkness. It was another text message from Alastair. 'When can I get the passes?' he asked. We finally got to the Meridien hotel at about two in the morning, had a nightcap and then turned in. Just before eight the next morning my phone rang. It was Campbell again. He was downstairs in reception. He wanted his tickets.

'Give me twenty minutes to get dressed,' I told him.

'I'm wearing an orange T-shirt,' he said.

'I know what you look like, Alastair,' I said.

He was in shorts and trainers having jogged his way over from the British ambassador's residence, where he was staying with his family. As we finally shook hands, I realised he'd been standing in a blast of air conditioning in a sweaty T-shirt, waiting for me.

In person, Campbell was immediately charming and chatty. We talked for ten minutes, he thanked me for the VIP passes and then, narrowing his eyes, he leaned forward and asked: 'Tell me, Jeremy — why is it that the French don't like Lance?'

Over the years, I have developed several answers to this question. Simon Barnes, chief sports writer on *The Times*, had asked me the same thing a couple of years earlier and then filed a piece highlighting French chauvinism that concluded: 'The French just don't like the cut of his jib.'

The reality was far more complicated than simply Lance's inability (and unwillingness) to charm his hosts. My usual responses to the 'why do they hate Lance' question ranged from 'because he's not French', 'because he makes it look too easy', 'because they like to think he's on drugs', 'because he can be a pompous ass' to 'because they're uncouth bigots'. Sometimes, it had been all of the above.

I paused for a moment, looked at Campbell and said: 'Maybe it's because they feel disconnected from him and don't really understand him, his culture or his attitude. They respect his achievement but I don't think they like him or warm to him. It's all the talk about him as a "brand". He's too much of a ready-made hero. That makes them suspicious. Tradition dictates that no rider should be bigger than the Tour itself, but these days that's happened with Lance.'

I told him about the way that Armstrong black-balled those who challenged him, like French rider Christophe Bassons and doping whistle-blower Filippo Simeoni, the Italian who had self-sabotaged his career by opting to testify against Ferrari: 'Some people feel that he was bullying Simeoni, that he was making his personal gripe more important than the Tour itself. Some say that he was taking control of a situation that wasn't his to take control of . . .'

Alastair Campbell listened intently, leaned in a little more, and then, with a wry smile, said: 'Hmm, yes – but I quite like that, you see . . .'

LEARNING THE HARD WAY

Message boards pulse with the poisonous, fetid glee of anonymous, untraceable hate. They post their rage in pixels, little darts of fury, for all to see. They hate Greg LeMond for his jealousy, his bitterness, for his attempts to debunk Lance Armstrong, Floyd Landis and Tyler Hamilton.

They hate Greg LeMond for believing that Americans could cheat or lie.

Greg LeMond – what did he ever do, compared to Lance? Why, he's even got a French name . . . What a Judas, what a turncoat.

And it's true: LeMond is deeply outraged by cycling's slew of doping scandals. He doesn't hide it and he tells anybody who cares to ask him exactly how he feels. But he also doesn't care if the dopers are Italian, French, British or American – it disgusts him. He belongs to a more genteel time in cycling, that, if not Corinthian, at least had some notion of etiquette and hands-across-the-ocean social responsibility.

And *shh . . . shoot!* No swearing, please honey.

There's one big difference between LeMond and Lance: Greg actually quite likes the French. He gets on with them. He rode for French sponsors, he speaks French well, he respects the differences and the traditions. In fact, he embraces them. He says his favourite French village is Venasque, tucked away at the foot of Mont Ventoux, with its slumbering mediaeval streets, old-fashioned bar-tabac and nearby olive groves and vineyards.

But all that old stuff, the cobbles, the morning bread ritual, the endless handshakes, the three-hour lunches, the multiple national holidays, the *bonjours*, and the *ça vas* – that's the stuff that makes Lance mad because it slows things down and gets in the way.

It is easy to see how LeMond became alienated from the new generation of cycling obsessives, the evangelical Lance fans. As Armstrong became more famous, LeMond kept on shooting him down, dividing opinion, pricking consciences, fuelling suspicion. Some said that he'd grown bitter and isolated, twisted by his own disappointments into attacking those who have come in his wake. Others see him as a failed romantic, an idealist, generally sickened by what has become of the sport he once loved.

But then a sense of fair play seems to be in LeMond's blood. His mother was a big fan of the Olympic Games, his sister a national-level gymnast. LeMond's parents instilled in him the belief that cheating and stealing was cheating and stealing from yourself: in the LeMond household, he recalls, cheating was 'just plain wrong'.

Yet Greg LeMond knows well enough that there has been no golden age in cycling's ethics. 'Through all the years of cycling there has always been unethical behaviour, a willingness to go one step further. But I came from a background with no history of the doping culture in cycling. I didn't even believe that it existed!'

He was eighteen when, riding for the American national team, he first came to Europe to race. 'I won against professionals, East Germans – strong countries.' That success led to a contract with the Renault team in the early 1980s. But even then, a boy racing against men, LeMond maintains that he remained an innocent abroad.

'This is not everybody else's perspective. I know other riders who were in different teams where there was obviously a doping culture. In a way, I kept my blinkers on . . . I purposely didn't want to go there. It would have shattered my ambitions in cycling.'

Unlike some others, Greg was lucky with his coaches. There was Cyrille Guimard, team manager at Renault and Bernard

Hinault's coaching guru, and then, following LeMond's move to La Vie Claire, Swiss sports scientist Paul Koechli. When Greg left Renault to join Hinault's new La Vie Claire team, Guimard was unimpressed. 'He implied that I would probably never win the Tour without him, and in my mind he meant that I would have to take "stuff" to win the Tour.'

LeMond says that Guimard's veiled but disparaging comment sealed his fate. 'I don't like to be held prisoner by anybody, or depend on them for my own success.' LeMond was fortunate in that Koechli was staunchly anti-doping and convinced that, with the right preparation, LeMond could win the Tour – and win it clean. Koechli's stance fuelled Greg's idealism even further. As a result, he remained isolated from what was going on around him.

'If you're an alcoholic you know a lot of other alcoholics,' LeMond says. 'Same if you're a drug addict. If you aren't in that crowd, you don't realise who's doing it and who isn't.'

In La Vie Claire's studious Koechli, he found a kindred spirit. 'Greg did not use any stuff,' Koechli maintained, in clipped English, years later. 'I say that two hundred per cent certain.' Both Koechli and LeMond believed that a reliance on doping was down to a lack of strength of character.

Yet despite the fine words and high ideals, LeMond was a professional cyclist racing in Europe: inevitably, he came to a crossroads, a point at which doping seemed seductive. Accidentally shot in a freak hunting accident in the spring of 1987, just a few months before he was due to defend the Tour title he had won in 1986, Greg almost bled to death. His comeback proved long and traumatic. For months on end, his form remained woeful.

Like other riders, he arrived at a watershed when he was at his most vulnerable, desperate for results, making his way back from injury, keen to justify himself to his sponsor. But he stepped back from the precipice.

LeMond went on to win two more Tours – in 1989 and 1990

– but as he entered his thirties, he could see the writing on the wall. The landscape had changed. Riders who had once finished far behind him were now leaving him for dead on the mountain passes. Blood doping, and in particular the then undetectable EPO, was rewriting the form book in his sport.

'At first, I didn't say, oh, they're taking drugs – I just wondered if maybe I wasn't as good as I thought. And in the back of my mind, I was worried that the lead pellets still in my body from my hunting accident were hindering my performance.

'We're talking about a ten per cent increase in average speeds of the Tour,' he recalls. 'I look back to 1991 as the crossroads in EPO use, because in 1990 I wasn't even at my best, but in 1991 I was highly prepared – as well as I'd been since 1986, when I won.

'There were probably sixty or seventy guys that year on EPO. I looked at my team, who'd won the race overall the previous year, and the difference between us and the dopers got more and more pronounced as the race went on.'

As EPO culture took root, the *omerta* tightened its grip. The dependence of the peloton's key figures on each other, allied to the pressure to maintain the sport's status quo, became increasingly apparent.

Champions opted to race less and trained in secret, returning dramatically to the scene to win key events. LeMond, in contrast, often accused of basing his whole season on simply the Tour, rode many of the Spring Classics, the Giro d'Italia and, usually, the World Championships. The long absences of others were described as training 'microcycles', although it may also have been a way to perfect 'preparation' and avoid detection. Many such riders went on to become cycling royalty, with a long line of successes to their names. Slowly but surely, the use of EPO became an open secret.

Exhausted and embittered, LeMond cut a dejected figure at his final few races in 1994. EPO use, he had realised, was sweeping unchecked through his sport. Testosterone and amphetamines were now drugs for novices or idiots. Certainly, blood transfusions had been used in the past, but a new, more sophisticated, more professional era of blood doping, administered by highly paid experts and fuelled by advances in medical technology, had opened up. LeMond became deeply outraged by the unblinking acceptance of it.

'If you understand the physiology of cycling, you will know that at the end of three weeks of the Tour, your haematocrit has a descending value. Those who aren't on EPO can start off with a certain power output and a certain amount of haematocrit, of red blood cells. But by the end of the Tour, there's usually a decrease in the red blood cell count, which correlates to a five to ten, maybe twelve, per cent decrease in oxygen intake.'

When cumulative fatigue is such a huge factor, EPO comes into its own. 'Certain riders would have a serious drop in haematocrit, perhaps from forty-three per cent to thirty-eight per cent. Now, imagine you're competing against an EPO user topping himself up to maybe fifty per cent, which, by all accounts in the mid 1990s was relatively low. Red blood cells correlate very closely to power output.

'When you take the spread between a guy whose level drops to thirty-eight per cent, compared to a guy who's racing at fifty-five per cent, and then run that over a three-week race – where the difference becomes increasingly pronounced – no matter how talented the first rider is, there's no way he's able to compete against the guy who's taking EPO. It's not about recovery,' he says. 'It's about getting the edge to win.'

By the mid 1990s, doctors were on the road with almost every leading team, supposedly keeping athletes healthy, guarding against doping by keeping their charges on the straight and narrow. For a while, baffled by the jargon of sports science, everybody fell for it: meanwhile, behind closed doors, blood was being manipulated and results perverted.

At the Telekom team of Bjarne Riis, Erik Zabel and Jan

Ullrich, institutionalised doping took the German squad to victory in the Tour in 1996. LeMond had seen it coming and after the disappointment of the 1991 Tour, he never again threatened to win a major race.

Even so, his image, that of a rare, clean winner of the Tour, has come under attack in recent years, perhaps because he is so vociferously anti-doping that he has sometimes sounded holier-than-thou. But he argues in his own defence that even at eighteen and nineteen, his results were outstanding. 'You'd have to believe that I was on drugs then, because my results were immediately at a high level – I was competitive against Hinault, the Tour de France champion. I was third in my first Tour. I showed consistency. There were no abnormally bizarre performances beyond my normal genetic level.'

But how does he respond to those who say that he is just bitter and jealous? Aren't the top riders faster now than twenty years ago simply because of better equipment and advances in training and physiology?

'Whenever I hear anybody say the training's better, the bikes are better . . . my career spanned fourteen years and probably the biggest innovations happened in the 1980s. Carbon fibre, aero bars, disc wheels, clipless pedals – that all happened when I was racing.'

He struggled to recover his form after his hunting accident, but puts that down to chronic anaemia, which he admits was treated during the 1989 Giro d'Italia with three iron shots. 'But I watched the doctor break open the vial in front of me. There was none of this "Oh, I'll come back in a minute with a syringe . . ." But people will say what they want about me . . . and that's one of the reasons I am so disgusted with the sport right now, because the riders in today's world taint anyone who's won the Tour in the past. If I had taken three illegal injections, why would I have ever said anything about them?'

★　　★　　★

When Greg LeMond retired, he left a vacuum in American cycling. Lance Armstrong soon filled it. LeMond, however, was not impressed. Greg and Lance, the traditionalist and the upstart, became rivals for the affections of the growing army of state-side cycling fans. Theirs was always an uneasy relationship, but they were tied together by their mutual business interests. By the turn of the millennium, fuelled by Armstrong's success, interest in road cycling in America was reaching unprecedented levels. Trek bikes, who sponsored Armstrong and who also distributed Greg's own LeMond-branded machines, were experiencing phenomenal sales.

On the back of that, a growing market for luxury cycling tours in France and Italy, tailored to silver-haired CEOs from California and New England, began to show itself. Trek Travel, another of the bike manufacturer's brand extensions, was quick to realise the opportunity.

Fronting it all was the lure of the Armstrong brand, the kick-ass legend that fuelled the dreams of each and every one of the corporate gurus as they pedalled their way through the Alps and Pyrenees in US Postal replica kit.

But then Greg LeMond would open his big mouth, butting in with some other inappropriate comment. As the 2001 race ended with a third Armstrong victory, a race in which he had climbed to victory on Alpe d'Huez ten minutes faster than Hinault and LeMond in 1986, Greg was asked by David Walsh what he thought of Lance's relationship with Ferrari.

'All I said was that I was disappointed,' LeMond recalls. 'And who wouldn't be? This was a sport that was trying to clean up and the guy who's won the Tour is calling Ferrari his best buddy. It just didn't make sense.'

Then he waited for the backlash.

Within forty-eight hours of Lance's victory, Greg and I were walking through Mayfair towards our lunch with the oil company. The next day, after Greg's flight landed back in the States, he switched on his phone. That was when Lance called.

It wasn't to ask if he'd picked up anything special in Harvey Nichols.

Greg and Kathy LeMond have claimed that Lance was threatening and aggressive – but Armstrong has dismissed this and asserted that LeMond was rambling and incoherent.

Lance wanted Greg to retract his comments about Ferrari. He refused, even though he enjoyed a business relationship with Trek, Armstrong's influential key sponsors, and was putting himself at risk. In the end, through a clumsily worded press release that saw the light of day a few weeks later, he apparently did. Like many others, I was stunned to see the retraction. It didn't sound like the Greg LeMond I knew. Knowing the depth of his feeling, I called him.

'What happened?' I asked him.

'They put a gun to my head,' LeMond said at the time. He still stands by that comment.

'Yeah, they did,' Greg says. 'I was under incredible duress from the whole Armstrong camp and my whole business was at stake.'

LeMond says that the press release, disowning his earlier comments to Walsh, came straight out of Lance Armstrong's office, through his agent, Bill Stapleton. 'I didn't even sign off on it. I just said, "Fuck it – do what you have to do. I'm off to Montana, I can't stand this."'

Enraged at the time, LeMond now finds Armstrong's defensive tactics amusing. 'Lance set the template on how to be the master of spin. Convince everybody there's a conspiracy, convince everybody that it couldn't be him, that it's always somebody else, that it's got to be a conspiracy against the Americans.'

But as Lance's popularity and power mushroomed, LeMond became increasingly withdrawn. He steered clear of the hate mail he attracted on message boards, but remained conscious of the anger that some felt towards him.

'People keep saying I don't have anything positive to say about American riders. Well, why should I? Why should I have to be a supporter just because they're Americans? I support the riders who speak out, I support the riders who come clean, who say this sport needs to be cleaned up because I don't want my sixteen-year-old kid racing in cycling.'

In April 2008, the Trek and LeMond relationship finally came to an end.

THE VALLEY OF THE TROLLS

*'Fucking trolls!' he said . . . Others might have been tempted to
ignore the trolls, or at least pretend to ignore them, but not
Armstrong. He watched them obsessively, getting ready to fight,
to go to battle, to take the bastards on.*

Daniel Coyle, *Lance Armstrong: Tour de Force*

It is wintertime in Britain. The sludge brown earth of
Cambridgeshire is as far from the humid scrubland of the Texas
Hill Country as is imaginable. The ground is barren and wet.
Fog swirls in across the fens and flatlands, slowing motorways
to a crawl and grounding flights across south-east England.

On a Sunday morning, the trolls' witch-finder general stands
on the touchline of a windswept football pitch, exhorting a
bunch of kids to greater efforts. David Walsh, back from yet
another trip, is at home near Cambridge. He is this football
team's coach and, since 2001, the king of the Lance Armstrong
sceptics, the torch bearer of the 'witch-hunt'.

After the confrontation in Pau, Walsh published two unflat-
tering books on Armstrong. The most recent, *LA Officiel* (2006),
was the sequel to the best-selling *LA Confidentiel* (2004). As
before, it was co-authored with former *L'Equipe* journalist Pierre
Ballester.

Once, back in the days when EPO use in the peloton was
still just a rumour, the American had been the subject of an
admiring portrait in Walsh's 1993 book, *Inside the Tour de France*.
But *Inside the Tour de France* is to the two *LA* books what *The
Sound of Music* is to *The Exorcist*.

Amid all the celebration of Armstrong the hero, Walsh became a consistent voice of dissent. Since 2001, the pair have fought their battle in flurries of legal activity in Britain, France and America. Like a brawl in the street, their battle for supremacy was an ugly but fascinating sight.

'He is the worst journalist I know,' the Texan said generously of the award-winning Irishman. And surely, the most bloody-minded.

Walsh just wouldn't let it lie, while Lance was hardly one to back down. In some ways they were more like each other than perhaps they realised. Much of their time seemed to be dedicated to getting mad – and getting even. Plotting the downfall of others is stressful and exhausting, bad for the soul, yet they both seemed to relish it. Armstrong never failed a drugs test and has always denied the use of performance-enhancing products. He never tires of pointing out his long track record of negative test results. When the *Sunday Times* published material from *LA Confidentiel*, Armstrong sued the paper and David Walsh for libel. He won.

Walsh has some allies but they are less powerful than Armstrong's. At first Walsh had the upper hand, but as things heated up, Walsh found his credibility under attack over the articles he authored questioning Armstrong's ethics.

But perhaps what the purist Walsh disliked most about Lance was the fact that he reversed the roles of the Tour and the Tourist; he flung tradition back at the French by debunking the notion that no rider is bigger than the Tour itself.

Yet even this is a myth. What of his French hosts? Armstrong's success was warmly embraced by the Tour, French television and even the hoteliers and restaurateurs of the hexagon who somehow put their misgivings to the back of their minds as the dollars rolled in. Only when Armstrong had retired from racing in July 2005 did they suddenly voice their concern. Armstrong exploited the Tour and in much the same way that the Tour had always used the riders, the old race exploited him.

For the most part, he deserved his bad press. Armstrong had his ways of controlling the media and he could be cunning. On the pretence of according an interview, Lance, through his press officer or other journalists, would obtain home or mobile phone numbers of his critics and call them unexpectedly, out of the blue, before launching into bitter tirades.

'It's Lance. You won't need your pen,' the Texan would hiss at a hapless journalist, cooking Sunday lunch for his family, before launching into an expletive-peppered denouncement of his work. At the same time he revelled in reminding them of his status, of how much they relied on his name to sell magazines or newspapers. '*Waddya gonna do when I'm gone?*' he'd taunt in his inimitable growl. On the few occasions that failed, he became increasingly confrontational. But he never backed down.

Towards the end of his final Tour, as I stood in a finish-line huddle with Johan Bruyneel, there was a lull in the conversation, which had turned towards the irritating detail that, despite his domination, Lance had yet to win one of that year's stages.

'You know that some French people are saying, given that it's his final Tour, that maybe Lance should throw caution to the wind, try to win a stage and show a little more panache . . .' I suggested.

Bruyneel snorted in derision. 'Panache, panache! I think winning seven Tours is enough panache!' My old mate Andy Hood, standing alongside, guffawed in amusement.

Two days later in Saint-Etienne, Lance was midway through his final press conference when my ears suddenly pricked up as he answered a question unrelated to panache (or my suggestion of his lack of it) by turning it into another diatribe against his critics.

'You know, some guy shoves a microphone in Johan's face and says, "he doesn't have any panache − where's the panache?"' he said, eyes scanning the pressroom, a threatening edge to his voice. 'Seven Tours gives you panache.'

A few rows ahead of me, I heard Hood's familiar guffaw once more.

In a sport that had never had a star of his status before,

belittling his critics was a tactic that worked well for Lance; some journalists, terrified of finding themselves on the blacklist, ostracised by the biggest star they had ever known, wilted in the full force of the Texan hairdryer.

But this was hardly Sir Alex Ferguson and the BBC. Lance's hectoring and secretive behaviour only fuelled the suspicion that he had something to hide. His lack of transparency, his control freakery, highlighted by his woeful relations with the European media, worked against him. Isolated in his tower of perfection and obsessed with winning, winning, winning, the whispering got louder and it made him madder than ever – madder than hell.

And winning, year after year, didn't seem to help. In fact, the more Lance won, the angrier he got. By the end of the 2005 Tour, Lance seemed very angry indeed. He couldn't even leave the Champs-Elysées without launching into another rant against the sceptics, although he spared the crowds in Paris the four-letter words. Like Michael Schumacher, whose unsmiling domination of Formula 1 only served to make him less popular each year, the Texan's po-faced persona did little for his relations with the Tour's homeland.

Walsh had homed in on this sentiment amongst the French, fuelling the notion that Armstrong Inc. had raped and pillaged the Tour and that all that would be left afterwards would be the wreckage of his dominion. The content of *LA Confidentiel*, in particular, stirred up a hornet's nest.

In 2004, the fuss about the book pricked the interest of SCA Promotions, a stateside risk insurance company. SCA Promotions, who provide what has been described as 'risk coverage for promotional contests', had been poised to send Armstrong a cheque for $5 million – his share of a bonus scheme taken out across three companies and worth, in total, $10 million. But then company president Bob Hamman started reading Walsh's and Ballester's damned book.

SCA became curious because they wished to explore the

possibility that Armstrong had used performance-enhancing drugs to win six Tours – and to cash in on what was effectively a bet he had made on himself. John Bandy, one of SCA's legal team, confirmed that payment was delayed because Hamman wanted to follow up some of the claims made by Walsh and Ballester in *LA Confidentiel*.

Initial media coverage of the case was deemed less than flattering by Armstrong, so through Bill Stapleton's offices at the CSE agency, he issued a statement, in which the standards and reputation of the French anti-doping laboratory at Châtenay-Malabry were relied upon.

Armstrong's statement, reproduced here in its entirety, set out his case:

Austin, Texas, 25 September

CSE is issuing the following statement in response to widespread media reports by CNN, the Associated Press and *USA Today* containing false and reputation-threatening information by SCA. This information pertains to the terms of an incentive bonus insurance policy with SCA on behalf of Lance Armstrong. The US Postal Service (USPS) Team, which Lance Armstrong leads, is jointly owned and managed by CSE and Tailwind Sports.

CSE is shocked and disappointed by public statements being made by SCA regarding this situation. Lance's record-setting six consecutive Tour de France victories, along with his inspirational story of cancer survivorship, is one of the greatest comeback stories of our day. With this achievement comes reward, including an incentive bonus structure common in the sports business. Lance's bonus structure was put in place in 2001 by his team to incent him to win six Tours de France, all in a row. At the time, the idea seemed far-fetched: he had only won two, and he had to win four more to get this year's bonus of $10 million. The bonuses were insured by three companies, one of which is SCA, a Dallas-based company that is responsible for $5 million of the payment to Lance. The insurance agreement is simple and clear: if Lance achieves six victories, he is paid his performance award. There is simply no question about the 'validity' of Lance's victory, and it has been confirmed by the organisers of the Tour de France and by the Union Cycliste International (UCI), the international governing body of cycling. SCA's failure to pay the final instalment of its bonus incentive insurance policy is a shameless and baseless breach of contract. Lance's 2002 and 2003 performance awards were insured under the same contract and, upon his victories, the sums were paid by SCA as required.

An SCA attorney's quote in *USA Today* stating 'We've requested drug test [results] to disprove the allegations — clean test results that should be easily attainable' is simply untrue and not supported by the facts.

Contrary to SCA's disingenuous and self-serving quote in *USA Today*, SCA is not interested in valid and authenticated 'testing results'; to the contrary, SCA, before considering payment, demanded free and unlimited access to 'every medical record and medical provider of Mr Armstrong; his complete medical history; all records of all Armstrong's past bonus awards; and all contracts involving Armstrong, Tailwind, US Postal Service, Capitol Sports & Entertainment, Disson Furst, and all related entities and individuals.' Even if SCA did have any legitimate interest in the drug and doping test results, ninety per cent of what SCA has demanded would have no relevance and further reveals the falsity of its statements. The actual testing protocols, consisting of fifty-two detailed pages, and the results of those tests were provided to SCA over a month ago.

On 16 August, 2004, CSE provided SCA CEO, Bob Hamman, with a letter from the UCI, which administered and enforced the anti-doping regulations and testing for the

Tour de France, authenticating Lance's clean testing record at the 2004 Tour de France. In the letter sent to SCA by the UCI's anti-doping manager, Christian Varin, he stated:

'I confirm that Mr Lance Armstrong was tested several times and all of the laboratory results were negative. I would also point out that the tests are performed in collaboration with the French Ministry of Sport. The laboratory is a "WADA accredited" [World Anti-doping Agency] laboratory [Châtenay-Malabry]. This year, we proceeded to urine anti-doping tests and blood anti-doping tests. Mr Armstrong was submitted to both kinds of tests. Also, all the test results are managed by another French independent body: The CLPD [Conseil de Lutte et de Prevention du Dopage] according to French legislation. As a conclusion, I reiterate the fact that Mr Lance Armstrong was tested several times and that all results were negative.'

Needless to say CSE is puzzled by SCA's accusations when we not only documented testing validation from the UCI over a month ago, but provided contact information and access to Mr Varin and the organisations that developed, applied and analysed the tests. Lance has made it unambiguously clear over the years that he does not use, nor has he ever used, performance-enhancing drugs. The baseless and mean-spirited doping allegations against Lance are not supported by any facts. He has been tested more than any other professional athlete in the world and has never failed a drug test.

Unfortunately, it appears that SCA is changing the rules when it is time to fulfil its obligation. The SCA website states: 'The concept behind Performance Coverage is simple: offer a professional athlete a cash bonus for an outstanding performance. When the athlete meets the stated mark, SCA funds the bonus in full and promptly.' We met our 'mark', and the bonus should be promptly paid – as advertised.

★   ★   ★

The Paris laboratory cited here as a model of efficiency is the same French laboratory that in 2005 'leaked' evidence fuelling allegations of EPO use by Armstrong in 1999 and that in 2006 returned two positive testosterone tests for his former teammate Floyd Landis. It is the same laboratory that Armstrong once described as having an 'excellent reputation'. Yet both Armstrong and Landis have now questioned the Châtenay-Malabry lab's ethics, competence and professionalism.

September 2004 was a busy month for Armstrong and his lawyers. In the same week, he opened proceedings against David Walsh and the *Sunday Times* and against SCA Promotions in the United States in pursuit of payment. The action against SCA Promotions was filed in Dallas by Lance and Tailwind Sports, the management company that owned his team, which, at that time was still sponsored by US Postal Service. Both cases were settled in Armstrong's favour. But Walsh and Ballester persisted. Armstrong's legal team said that the claims in *LA Confidentiel* were groundless and pointed to his long run of negative tests, both in and out of competition. Meanwhile, SCA hired private investigators, and with a ruling not expected for up to eighteen months, began turning over rocks to see what they could come up with. This forced some of Lance's former confidants, such as Frankie Andreu, to choose sides.

Walsh's campaign against Armstrong made him the black sheep of the press corps. Suddenly, he found that friends were hard to come by. When we spotted the Irishman trudging his way around Liège on his own as the 2004 Tour started, we joked as we sped past that this was because nobody wanted to be seen car-sharing with the troll king by Lance's spies.

Incredibly, this turned out to be true.

So paranoid had Armstrong made other journalists that Walsh became a virtual exile. The combined efforts of Lance and The Entourage, his team manager Johan Bruyneel and US Postal's press officer, Jogi Muller, aided by some press-room cronies, strong-armed others, clearly of little resolve, into distancing Walsh.

If Walsh was spotted travelling or even talking with other journalists, Muller would scuttle back to Lance and Bruyneel. Armstrong wanted us to choose between his way and the highway. Being responsible international sports journalists with high-minded ethics, most of us just sat on the fence.

With Armstrong's popularity at its peak, few who worked in cycling could afford to be blacklisted, and those who maintained their friendship with Walsh were tarred with the same brush. On one occasion, journalist Rupert Guinness and Bruyneel almost came to blows, when the Australian was reprimanded for being too friendly to Walsh. Guinness, one of Lance's close confidants in the early years when he had taken his first uncertain steps in Europe, was disgusted. He too became *persona non grata* in the Armstrong camp.

Towards the end of his career, if Armstrong and his associates had been able, they would surely have printed the same press release in every newspaper and magazine. His inability to achieve total control made Armstrong increasingly surly, although his face lit up when a TV camera turned his way. Printed media he could do without, but moving pictures he loved.

That was reflected by his choice of press officer. The hapless Jorg 'Jogi' Muller was ill-equipped for the job. An unremarkable ex-professional, Muller spoke many languages, but showed little understanding of the subtleties of the press. Once, I emailed him a simple query on the status of Lance's relationship with Sheryl Crow. 'I know nothing,' came the reply.

On another occasion, when Armstrong's paranoia was at its height, Muller forcefully tried to persuade a leading American sports writer to hand over a tape of a conversation she and other journalists had had with Walsh. Stapleton and Armstrong scrambled to apologise.

Muller's ability to say no to all requests became legendary, as did his inability to remember a name. Eventually, I became firmly established on the blacklist although I don't think that Muller, with characteristic vagueness, really knew why. Somebody —

Lance or Stapleton, or maybe Bruyneel – had just told him to add my name to it.

At the same time, Muller blithely continued his own business association with Michele Ferrari, even after the Italian was convicted of doping offences (although Ferrari was later acquitted following an appeal). Muller, while blocking yet another interview request with Armstrong, would at the same time use his contacts with the media to promote the website 53x12.com – an online training consultancy he had set up with Ferrari.

'Sorry,' he'd say. 'Lance is not available – but can I send you an email about my new website?' Muller unashamedly publicised his relationship with the Italian even as Armstrong again defended himself against allegations of doping. Given that he was responsible for Armstrong's relationship with the press, it was bizarre behaviour.

The Swiss-German also led the increasingly creative bad-mouthing of those who spoke out against Armstrong. He had strong support from Armstrong's two press-room stooges, whose meal ticket was their 'special' relationship with the Tour champion. The pair would squabble over which of them was closest to the Texan. I have always had a sneaking feeling that Lance secretly enjoyed this. Conversations with the stooges debating the merits of the latest allegations against Armstrong invariably ended the same way. One by one, they would shoot down Lance's critics. The French? 'They're lazy.' David Walsh? 'He's a crazy obsessive!' Greg LeMond? 'He's washed-up and jealous!' Filippo Simeoni? 'A liar and a proven drugs cheat.'

It was remarkably easy to fuel the galloping paranoia of The Entourage. In the aftermath of David Millar's two-year ban, I asked Johan Bruyneel if – given that Dave's old mate Lance had been such a shoulder to cry on during the dark days of his drugs bust – the Belgian and his Texan team leader might consider signing Millar for US Postal once his ban had been served.

Bruyneel frowned. 'Yes, somebody told me you'd started that rumour,' he said.

I laughed in disbelief. 'Maybe you shouldn't believe all the gossip you hear, Johan,' I said. Two years later, Bruyneel was scrabbling to sign Ivan Basso.

Exchanges like this guaranteed my place on the blacklist. But then by 2005, more of us were on it than not. Bruyneel, Muller and Armstrong had become so despised for their hostility towards the press that we wore blacklist status like a badge of honour.

Ultimately, Armstrong's never-ending suspicions became a self-fulfilling prophecy. By the time he had won his final Tour, he certainly had enemies. After half a decade spent defending himself, he was so paranoid that every encounter became claustrophobic, heavy with suspicion. But then my feeling was that, isolated in his control tower, he wouldn't have wanted it any other way. There was now a stream of ostracised confidants; the journalists were bad enough, but then there were the embittered and resentful ex-pros queuing up to knife him, the former personal assistants demanding money, as well as – with breathtaking hypocrisy – the Tour de France directors who had fallen at his feet as the dollars rolled in.

By the end of the seven-year reign, it wasn't just the French who felt that Armstrong had long outstayed his welcome. The notion, so eloquently expressed in Daniel Coyle's excellent book, *Lance Armstrong: Tour de Force*, that despite all the money, cars, women and houses, Lance was secretly lonely and isolated, took root as his 'friends' turned on him. It was time for him to climb out of the bear pit.

PROTECTING THE INTERESTS
OF THE PELOTON

The 2004 Tour de France is one day away from the Champs-Elysées.

Lance Armstrong, taut and lean in the yellow jersey, strides down the central aisle of the Besançon media centre into the Tour winner's press conference. A ripple of applause splutters into life, initiated by the American media contingent. When it is not picked up by the Europeans present, it fades away.

Armstrong, followed by The Entourage, strides purposefully towards the platform and the waiting bank of microphones and cassette recorders. Cameras flash, tapes whirr. He sits down. The questions begin.

Lance's drawl booms out of the PA, easy, relaxed and assured. There is no Kimmage or Walsh out there, no inquisitor to face. He had dominated the Tour to secure his sixth win. Once again he has put them all in their place. The naysayers and sceptics among the media and his rivals – where are they now? After six years, Armstrong's supremacy was complete. His multimillion dollar fund-raising efforts through his cancer foundation, the sweeping success of the Livestrong wristbands, his celebrity profile and the successful rebuttal of any attacks on his reputation, had made him appear almost untouchable. Even his bitterest critics had to admit that he was an extraordinary human being. Lance's legendary status now transcended his sport: for many people, his good deeds – the fund-raising, the campaigning for better cancer treatment, the hope he offered the hopeless – nullified any concerns there may have been over his effect on his sport. How could somebody who had done so much for others be anything but a force for good?

So as he sits down in Besançon, there is a stalemate, a predictability, in the air. Nonetheless, my tape recorder runs, just in case. I stand up, stretch my legs and stroll around to the side of the low stage. The questions continue; he smiles, shrugs, jokes, bats them back. I walk around to the rear of the stage. Double doors are open to the car park and a warm breeze wafts in. The US Postal liveried station wagon with blacked-out windows is parked beyond the threshold.

Lance's bodyguard stands there in the doorway, waiting.

'Last question please,' says US Postal's press attaché, Dan Osipow. His master's voice echoes once more around the hall. Then, job done, Lance is on his feet, making his way through the tangle of wires and speakers. He steps down from the back of the stage for the short walk to the waiting car. His minders are lagging behind as he strides towards the doors.

From under the brim of his baseball cap, he clocks me. I see a flicker of recognition but he keeps walking, keeps looking straight ahead. I take a step forward. He adjusts his cap.

Before I realise it's happened, he's past me and out through the doors, into the evening sunshine and a throng of adulation.

In the 2004 Tour, Armstrong was more dominant than he had ever been. He won by six minutes, he won six stages, he sneered at the boo boys, he hobnobbed with George W. Bush and John Kerry. He kissed Sheryl Crow. He drank Château de Fieuzal 1998 when victory was assured. He flung his supremacy in the face of his critics. Even as the doping scandals clouding the achievements of lesser riders multiplied, he remained the Tour's feudal king.

There was, however, one thing that displeased him: an Italian rider, Filippo Simeoni, who had testified against Michele Ferrari in an Italian courtroom and who continued to speak out against doping. Armstrong brushed him aside. 'He is like a child killing ants,' observed former French professional Laurent Jalabert, during the Tour. And it wasn't the first time that Armstrong had invoked the power of the *omerta* to assert his authority.

During the 1999 Tour, French professional Christophe Bassons had endured a brief feud with Armstrong. The Frenchman, then twenty-five, was riding for the La Française des Jeux team, a contract he'd secured after leaving the Festina team. When Festina had crashed and burned twelve months earlier, even his shamed teammates had universally acknowledged that Bassons was an intransigent non-doper.

That status ensured his notoriety. In a column he was writing for *Le Parisien*, in July 1999, Bassons questioned the ethics of the peloton and insisted that doping was still a significant problem. When he heard what Bassons had said, Armstrong, heading towards his remarkable first victory, sought him out. Armstrong later confirmed that, in a brief mid-race conversation, he had told Bassons that what he was saying was not good for the sport and that maybe, if he was so disenchanted with cycling, he should seek another profession. Bassons agrees with the gist of this account, but his version of the exchange is more blunt.

'Lance said, "Why don't you fuck off?"' Bassons recalled.

The encounter with Armstrong proved catastrophic for Bassons' career. Within hours some colleagues were ignoring him, while others implored him to keep his mouth shut. Even his own team manager, Marc Madiot, these days a voluble proponent of clean sport and leading light in the Movement for Credible Cycling, rounded on him. It was too much for Bassons and he quit the Tour in a shattered and distraught state. His career never truly recovered. Bassons moved to Bordeaux to work for the French Ministry for Sport and Culture.

Six years later, history repeated itself. At the 2004 Tour, Lance tackled a second whistle-blower.

Filippo Simeoni was a lowly Italian rider, best known for a stage win in the Tour of Spain, at which his maverick streak had first showed itself. As he rode towards victory and entered the final hundred metres, he stopped short of the finish and then walked across the line, triumphantly carrying his bike above his head. Later, he claimed this gesture was in tribute to the victims of the 9/11 terrorist attacks and in support of world peace. Showing their usual indulgence of rider eccentricities, the UCI fined him heavily.

Simeoni's unconventional behaviour was long forgotten by July 2004 when he raced in the Tour de France for the Domina Vacanze team. Established as a very able *domestique*, his presence at the Tour, riding in the same peloton as Armstrong, created a stir among the riders. He wasn't seen as a joke any more, but more as a loose cannon. He had spat in the soup in an Italian courtroom. He had broken the *omerta*.

Questioned by the Italian police as part of a detailed and comprehensive investigation into Michele Ferrari, Simeoni had agreed to testify. As Armstrong vigorously defended his relationship with Ferrari, Simeoni told the investigating judge that Ferrari had advised him on the use of banned substances, including EPO. He also confessed to doping himself.

Armstrong was enraged. Simeoni, he said, was not a credible witness. He described him as an 'absolute liar' in an interview in *Le Monde*. Few had imagined, however, that this bitter feud would be so publicly played out on the road during the Tour de France.

At first nothing happened. As he and Simeoni rode side by side in the peloton, Armstrong was at first merely dismissive towards the Italian, feigning a lack of interest in his presence. Then when Simeoni made plain his intention to win a stage, things got personal.

Simeoni escaped into a two-man breakaway on the ninth stage to Gueret: Armstrong and his team drove the pursuit. Simeoni and his breakaway companion, Inigo Landaluze, were overtaken by the main field just sixty metres from the finish line.

'We rode really strongly, really hard. It was amazing we got caught,' the Italian said afterwards.

He added that there were 'strange conversations' going on among the team cars, hinting that, even though they had no tactical interest in chasing Simeoni, Armstrong's US Postal team may have asked other team managers to get their riders to assist in the pursuit. Such an alliance would be usual if a contender for overall victory had been in the breakaway, or if Armstrong had suddenly become a top sprinter. Neither was the case.

For the next ten days, there was a truce: Simeoni did his job fetching and carrying for his team in the mountain stages, watching from a distance as Armstrong wrapped up another Tour win.

But when, on the humdrum eighteenth stage that began the journey north from the Alps towards Paris, Simeoni stole into another breakaway with five riders, the unthinkable happened: Armstrong, leading the Tour by a street, set off in lone pursuit. Once again, there was no tactical rationale to the American's behaviour. At that moment in the 2004 Tour, Lance had the race won and the Italian posed no threat to anyone – or so it seemed.

When he set off alone, in fierce pursuit of Simeoni, Armstrong was assured of final victory in the 2004 Tour. The Italian was languishing in 113th place, two hours and forty-two minutes behind him. But a stage win was up for grabs and like all the other *domestiques* in the race, with the Eiffel Tower looming on the horizon, Simeoni was desperate to bag one.

Armstrong, however, was not having it. He could see the headlines, the Ferrari questions in the press conference, the sudden renewal of interest in Simeoni's views on doping – *always doping*. So he slammed his feet down on the pedals and gave chase, hell-bent on stopping him.

If the main peloton was stunned by Armstrong's pursuit of Simeoni, the breakaway sextet were equally bemused when they saw the pair closing in on them. But they quickly realised that their hopes of staying clear to the finish were doomed with the *maillot jaune* in their number and the peloton obliged to chase. Unfortunately for Filippo, none of them had the courage to tell Lance to back off; instead, realising that the American had joined them seeking only to poison Simeoni's chances of a stage win, they turned on the Italian.

That afternoon, Filippo found himself shot by both sides; damned if he did, damned if he didn't. It was a defining moment both for him and for Armstrong. The Italian realised that he was now forever tainted as a professional cyclist, while the darker side of Lance's personality was revealed for all to see. Another rider might have told the Texan where to go and then ridden on regardless, but like Christophe Bassons before him, Filippo hesitated. Then, as peer pressure mounted, his resolve crumbled. Out of respect to the leading quartet, who after all, were seeking only to snatch some crumbs from the king's table, the Italian backed off.

Armstrong had achieved his goal. He had made it plain to his peers that Simeoni's decision to testify against Ferrari had made him *persona non grata* in professional cycling. The Italian could only watch despairingly as the breakaways powered ahead. Alone together in no-man's-land, as he and Lance freewheeled, waiting to be swallowed up by the chasing peloton, words were exchanged. Television cameras captured the moment, but remained out of earshot. Later, Simeoni alleged that Armstrong had issued threats and told him that it was a mistake to testify against Ferrari. Armstrong, he claimed, had told him, 'I have lots of time and lots of money. I will destroy you.'

A year later Armstrong expressed some regret. 'I made a mistake to go after him that day, but I never said the things he said I did.' But his words came too late to salvage Simeoni's career. When the main field did catch up to the pair, Simeoni endured a volley of abuse as rider after rider, including his Italian compatriots, taunted him. He slipped to the back of the field, fighting back tears. Armstrong claimed that several riders had congratulated him on his actions.

In a frank interview with journalist Daniel Friebe in 2004, Simeoni claimed that Daniele Nardello, a former Italian national champion, told him, 'You're a disgrace – you're spitting in the bowl you're eating from.' He claimed that other Italian riders – Filippo Pozzato, Andrea Peron and Giuseppe Guerini – picked up on that theme and also abused him.

After the stage finish, in Lons-le-Saunier, both Simeoni and Armstrong were interviewed live on French television.

Simeoni was tearful with rage. 'He showed today in front of the whole world what kind of person he is,' he said. 'It's a sin.'

Lance's response was enigmatic. 'I was protecting the interests of the peloton,' he said. 'All Simeoni wants to do is to destroy cycling and that's not correct. When I went back to the group they said *"chapeau"* – that's because they understand that this is their job and that they absolutely love it and they're committed to it and don't want somebody within their sport destroying it.' Simeoni was not to be allowed the oxygen of publicity that is the stage-winner's due.

That was not the end of it. On the final day of the race as the riders neared the Parisian suburbs, the feud resumed. Simeoni had been simmering with anger since the first confrontation. So he attacked again, this time deliberately, vengefully, raining on Lance's victory parade.

The opening kilometres of each Tour's final stage are a celebratory procession, given over to photo opportunities and mugging for the cameras. Riders swap bikes and parking cones are worn as hats – this kind of weary student jape passes for wit in the final hours of the Tour. In another clichéd tradition, the film crews and photographers mass around the winner as he poses with his teammates, holding aloft brimming champagne flutes.

But in 2004, just as Lance and his US Postal boys manoeuvred into position, fizz in hand, ready to pose for the cameras and toast a sixth successive victory, Filippo Simeoni decided to attack.

'I was so angry,' he said. 'Had I not done it, I couldn't have lived with myself. I thought: "I'll show you the victory parade to Paris." I waited until all of the photographers went to take Armstrong's photo and then – *boom!*'

Simeoni's bravado had a spectacular effect. To a chorus of shouting and swearing, half-empty champagne flutes were tossed away, motorbikes careered across the road in panic and shutters clicked manically as Armstrong and his team sprinted into action and gave pursuit. The attack did not last long but even then, perhaps because he realised that he would never get such an opportunity again, Simeoni had still not finished messing with Texas. Maybe he'd never seen the bumper stickers.

There was a lull. Then the Italian attacked again. In the press room, we laughed in disbelief and then cheered as the punch-drunk underdog, Simeoni, refused to stay down. He got back to his feet, ready to take more punishment.

But the final knockout was coming. Incredulous at the Italian's nerve, Lance and his 'blue train' saw red again – faces contorted with rage, they sped after him in muscular pursuit.

Metre by metre, Armstrong's team reeled Simeoni in as the convoy neared rue de Rivoli. When the peloton drew alongside, a shower of phlegm arched through the air towards him. It ran down his tanned legs as the peloton roared past. Simeoni – brave, naive . . . stupid, *stupid*, Filippo – was swallowed back into the field, only to be insulted once more by those whose dignity he was trying to defend.

This was cycling's law of silence – the hateful, oppressive *omerta* – made flesh.

MEETING BY THE RIVER

It is raining hard in Laval. In the November dusk, Saturday afternoon shoppers are scurrying home. Daniel Friebe and I cross the bridge over the river Mayenne and head for the main square. Rain runs down our necks. An old carousel stands under an avenue of palm trees, dripping in the downpour. In the gloom, we search for the Foyer Culturel on the allée du Vieux Saint-Louis. Meeting here, in this pretty but anonymous northern French town, are the gurus of doping dissent, the high priests of trolldom. Tonight's debate is the second in a series of occasional get-togethers in which France's cycling exiles and cynics talk through their experiences and affirm their solidarity against doping. Clutching a bottle of champagne – the media invitation asked that we arrived early bearing champagne and cake – we climb a rickety staircase to an upstairs annexe, set aside for the media to meet the speakers. We peer through the doorway.

There are perhaps twenty people in the room. I spot some berets, goatees and cravats. Are these people extras from a revival of *'Allo 'Allo*? 'Erm, you first then,' I instruct Daniel, a little ungallantly. We walk through the door . . . *et voila!* We join the French doping Resistance.

Apart from a handful of wives and girlfriends, those in the room are notorious enough to give Hein Verbruggen and Lance Armstrong chronic heartburn. On my right is Willy Voet, the former *soigneur* whose boot-load of drugs kick-started the Festina Affair in 1998. Voet, now a bus driver in the Alps, is chatting to his old boss, dapper Bruno Roussel, once Festina's team manager and architect of their pills-for-prizes wage structure, but now – oh, the irony! – an estate agent.

Orchestrating things and looking slightly baffled to see us, is Antoine Vayer, former trainer to the Festina team. Central to Vayer's loathing of the modern Tour is his belief that it is 'inhumane'. Through his constant, bitter critiques, Vayer long ago established himself as one of the leading sceptics of the Tour's efforts to clean itself up. He has been unfairly depicted as an arch-critic solely of Armstrong, but to give him his due, he in fact rails against cycling as a whole. He targets promoters and sponsors as well as individual riders and believes an amnesty is the only way to start afresh. He nailed his colours to the Troll mast by aligning himself with Walsh and Ballester in their two 'LA' books.

Across the room, Christophe Bassons, French cycling's *Monsieur Propre* (Mr Clean), is deep in conversation with former world mountain-biking champion and self-confessed doper, Jerome Chiotti, who renounced his world title in a very public epiphany. Bassons wears a wry smile, as if permanently amused by a private thought, which may be the realisation that it is now getting on for a decade since he crossed swords with Armstrong at the 1999 Tour; Chiotti, however, just looks bemused, much as he did on the day when, in front of the media, he lifted his gold medal over his head and disowned it.

Further away, Ballester and Walsh, chief architects of the supposed Armstrong 'witch-hunt', chat together with lawyer Thibault de Montbrial and French journalists Stephane Mandard and Benoit Hopquin, both of *Le Monde*, consistently the most outspoken anti-doping newspaper within France.

I haven't seen Ballester for a long time, hardly at all in fact since the 1999 Tour, when he crossed his own bridge to confirmed scepticism. I have always liked him, but he is now a little distant, different from the wry and funny journalist I met when I covered my first Tour. Lance had got on well with him too, giving him time on a regular basis, until he realised that Pierre had crossed to the other side. Ballester, like Walsh, has been through it. He left *L'Equipe*, not on the best of terms, soon after the 1999 Tour, when he had reported on Lance's first victory with an icy *froideur* that set him apart from much of the European media. Effectively, he had accused his press-room colleagues of complicity. Perhaps that is what now hangs in the air between us.

At the time, his scepticism was apparently unappreciated by his editors. Ironically, seven years later, he finally got the editorial support he'd deserved, when, in August 2005, *L'Equipe* published the infamous front-page splash, the *Mensonge Armstrong* (the Armstrong Lie), alleging that the Texan had used EPO during the 1999 Tour. Armstrong has repeatedly denied this.

Nearby, seated at a table, his partner by his side, is Laurent Roux, the former Tour 'King of the Mountains', once a true and celebrated goodfella, a 'made' guy, a rider who was, by his own admission, steeped in doping to the point of addiction. His catharsis, like that of Philippe Gaumont, was enforced by his arrest and trial. Roux has dealt drugs and served time. He is older, embattled, heavier set than the last time I saw him, and seems diminished and defeated by his life. In 2006, Roux was one of the key witnesses in a doping trial in Bordeaux. He was injecting himself with *pot belge* – a heady brew composed of amphetamines, caffeine, cocaine and heroin, that first came to light during the Festina Affair – several times a day. He also sold it to others. Depression and an eight-month prison sentence followed. Once up on the stage, Roux speaks rarely and hesitantly about how miserable his reliance on drugs made him.

'When you dope and you still don't win, then you just start taking more and more,' Roux says. Doping, I realise, is wonderful for those who win and get away with it, but a prison for those who dope and lose.

Walsh is listening but as he speaks little French, he sits focussing on some distant horizon, as around him the naysayers, bad boys and whistle-blowers – trolls one and all – rail against the evils of doping. Only the occasional mention of the heavily accented

A-word — '*Eurmstreuhng*' — snaps Walsh back to attention. The rest of the time, he is a weary and jet-lagged figure, listening distractedly as the grim testimonies to cycling's dysfunction continue.

So here they all are, denouncing the pillars of cycling's establishment, alongside Walsh: Bassons, Voet, Roussel, Ballester, Chiotti, Vayer — the high priests of scepticism — and me.

And me . . .

Does this make me one of them? Here, on a wet night in a nondescript town in rural France, have I finally — definitively — shifted off the fence, and crossed the bridge to the other side, taking my place alongside the nerdy naysayers, when I could be hanging with Cool Hand Lance, as he high-fives his way to another lucrative sponsorship deal?

I tell myself that I love cycling — *I still love cycling* — but, most of all, I suddenly understand, in the dim light of Laval's Foyer Culturel as Laurent Roux bows his head and confesses his sins and an unexpected wave of sadness washes over me, I hate doping and I hate the misery that goes with it.

Laurent Roux may have been ready to bare his soul, but there are not many present to witness his catharsis. The auditorium in Laval is only half full.

The people listening intently to Roux and Bassons, Voet and Roussel, are those who've braved the pouring rain and who care, *really* care, about being tricked and conned by dopers. When they open the debate to the floor, there are some poignant moments. An old man's voice trembles and he is close to tears when he stands up to question the panel, berating the journalists present for not being more combative and campaigning.

Bassons, a more hardened character now than the boyish and vulnerable rider who was bullied out of the 1999 Tour, offers the old man some hope. He is feisty and eloquent, emerging as a worthy spokesperson for a generation who did not want to dope, but who understood the inevitability of it. He is pragmatic about what cycling has put him through.

'I didn't care that there were riders more successful than me, but it was annoying that they didn't want to look at the real reasons why they were faster than me,' he says. 'I never wanted to be a big star or anything, because I enjoyed racing so much that the competition was enough. So I rode according to my own limits, to try and improve my performance. I raced against myself.'

Bassons agrees that the UCI's fifty per cent health-check test only exacerbated a dire situation and allowed doping to continue. It didn't prove the use of EPO, it was unfair to athletes with naturally high haematocrit, it labelled riders as dopers without providing concrete evidence of any wrongdoing, it didn't attack the trafficking or supply of illegal EPO – it was a red herring, a PR move, a Band-Aid when in fact major surgery was needed.

Bassons is energised enough to give those who want to listen a glimmer of hope, but as the small gathering files out onto the wet street, I wonder where are the rest of them? Have people given up? Have they admitted defeat? Have they become so accustomed to doping scandals that, when rider after rider makes a mockery of the Tour de France they can just, with a Gallic shrug, say *tant pis*?

A MATTER OF LIFE AND DEATH

In the Vendée region of western France, the 2005 Tour is about to begin. We wait in a humid aircraft hangar of a press room for the arrival of Lance Armstrong. Nearby sits Paul Kimmage, a ghost from the Tour's past, a former professional contemporary to Greg LeMond and Bernard Hinault. He seems uneasy. Restlessly and reluctantly, he is attending the start of the Tour on behalf of the *Sunday Times*.

Armstrong's control of the media was now so complete that few voices of dissent were heard. There was not to be a repeat of the Armstrong-Walsh showdown in Pau in 2001. By this stage of his career, Jogi Muller and his assistant, Mark Higgins, ensured that the microphone only ever reached friendly hands.

On the rare occasions that a 'difficult' question was asked – and by that I mean an inquisitor intrigued by Armstrong's ethics somehow managing to snatch the microphone – Muller and Higgins would spring into action. Muller would glare accusingly at the Tour's own press officials and Higgins would point his digital camera at the troll concerned, capturing his act of defiance.

Lance, realising that he was being questioned by one of the non-believers, would slowly fix his gaze on his inquisitor, with The Look, his 'Me? You question me? How *very* dare you!' glare on his face. Muller, Higgins and Johan Bruyneel, manager of Armstrong's new team, the Discovery Channel, would follow suit. Armstrong would pause, growl a one-line response and move on.

Eventually, there is a flurry of activity and Lance arrives. He confidently fields the opening questions. Then, unexpectedly, Kimmage puts his hand up. Discovery's media minders seem unsure as to who he is, until he opens his mouth, starts asking a question and suddenly everybody remembers what Paul Kimmage is best known for.

'Lance,' he says, 'has your preparation for the Tour de France changed in any way following the conviction of your performance consultant, Michele Ferrari, for sporting fraud?'

Lance's eyes narrow in recognition. *Ah, a troll.* Realising that he is being questioned by one of Walsh's acolytes – worse still, a smuggled-in, treacherous troll who used to be a pro – he turns his gaze on his inquisitor.

So, it's you, Kimmage . . .

Higgins presses the shutter on his digital camera and the muffled click fills the silence. Soon this troll will be filed along with the others. Bruyneel joins Lance in the glaring contest. The pro-Lance lobby turn, crane their necks and glare too. The long and meaningful pause ends.

'Absolutely . . . not,' growls Lance.

Another transatlantic voice piped up with another bland question on chateaux and wine and Kimmage's temerity was quickly forgotten. Later that day, as I rummaged in the boot of my car, I clocked Kimmage, boredom etched across his features, strolling aimlessly among the press cars and team buses.

'Hello, Paul,' I said. At that time, I believe I was still seen by him as complicit – soft on doping, soft on the causes of doping. But he was cordial enough. 'Enjoying yourself?' I asked.

'I can't wait to get out of here,' he said.

'Happy with that answer?' I asked, referring to Lance's response to his question.

'What d'you expect?' he shrugged.

'They took your picture,' I said.

'Do they do that all the time?' he asked.

'Only for the troublemakers . . . you should be honoured.'

I told him he should talk to Philippe Gilbert, the Belgian

rider who spoke openly about doping, suggesting he would make an interesting interviewee. Then, inevitably, we started to talk about David Millar.

Prior to the collapse of his career in the aftermath of the Cofidis scandal, Millar had refused Kimmage an interview, citing his whistle-blowing history as justification. Kimmage was still seething. I could see why. In response to Millar's rebuttal, Kimmage had sent him a copy of his pioneering book, *Rough Ride*, the first of cycling's confessionals.

'For Millar to have the nerve to say to me, "With your reputation . . ." *What the fuck is that?*'

'He's still a big kid,' I responded. 'I don't think he can cope with all this, he's out of his depth. He's too vulnerable to deal with all the shit in the sport.'

'You feel sorry for him, do you?' Kimmage said sharply.

'Erm, a little,' I said hesitantly. 'It's not like he planned it all. He's not a megalomaniac or control freak. David's chaotic. You said that you were a victim. Isn't David too?'

Kimmage's eyes narrowed. 'Yeah – and a very successful one at that,' he said.

After that, Paul Kimmage and I had unfinished business. I wanted to talk to him more, about his experiences during his transition from rider to journalist, and about his anger with Millar.

We met again at the end of 2006, in a café in St Christopher's Place, tucked away behind Oxford Street. Shoppers laden with bags sat hunched over lattes and hot chocolates as the uphill march towards Christmas continued. Kimmage was leaving it all behind, flying to Australia to report on the Ashes series. His Christmas lunch would be seafood and white wine, eaten under blue skies in sandals and shorts, far from the fog and frozen ground, the cancelled flights and motorway misery.

Kimmage has made a remarkable journey, from anonymity in the peloton to a feature writer on the *Sunday Times*. His journalistic career was built on the success of *Rough Ride*. The book details a naif's battle to retain his integrity – much to the scorn of all around him – and is one of the best sports books ever written. But in writing it, he had broken the *omerta* and *Rough Ride* ensured that, in cycling at least, Kimmage's name became a dirty word.

We order coffee. He tells me he's only agreed to meet me because of the tip I gave him about Philippe Gilbert. I explain what this book is about. He listens and then quickly takes me aback by saying that, ultimately, our journey has been the same. 'You invested your trust in the sport and it was betrayed. Like me.'

When, in 2006, Kimmage went back to the Tour, he covered the whole event. 'In a perverse sort of way I enjoyed it,' he says. 'But I'm pretty sure I won't go again, because I find it very hard to deal with people when I go back.'

Paul ran into some old acquaintances on the 2006 Tour. They were awkward encounters. It wasn't easy coming face to face with those who, in team cars and behind microphones, were propping up a system that he now despises and wants to tear down.

'Most of the guys I raced with I'm now on pretty good terms with, but when I see the status attributed to other people who are held up as icons, some of them complete and utter fucking liars, it really drives me crazy. I find that very difficult.'

He took his bike and rode in the Etape du Tour, the weekend warrior's race within the race, run over the route of one of the Tour's key stages, a few days before the pros tackle it for real.

'I love cycling, really love it,' he says. 'Absolutely. And I do love the Tour, it's a great event . . . but it's just a complete tragedy that it's been destroyed in that way.'

In a way, Kimmage's return to the Tour, documented in the *Sunday Times* – they could have called it '*Rough Ride II: No one likes him and he don't care*' – had a perfect ending. The climax of his three weeks on the 2006 Tour saw Floyd Landis' 'wonder' victory in Morzine, a win that has became infamous for the positive testosterone test that followed soon afterwards.

Even before Landis crossed the finish line alone after his marathon attack, Kimmage was shaking his head. 'I couldn't believe it. People I knew were jumping around like kids in sweet shops, but I thought it was complete bollocks. I don't know anybody who can recover from being as bad as that, to then killing everybody the next day, without recourse to doping.'

A week or so later, following the confirmation of his positive test, it was Landis whose name was mud. Kimmage says he got a kick out of that.

As a shy and puritanical young professional in Europe, Paul Kimmage felt the pressure for a long time before he succumbed to doping. Curiously, though, he does not regard himself as a doper.

'I doped three times, in three criterium races, races that were fixed. Tell me, what was the benefit of doing that? So I don't regard myself as ever having doped, although quite clearly I used amphetamines three times. In some ways it was a good thing to have done, because anybody who told me afterwards that the drugs didn't work, I'd just laugh at, because they transformed me.'

But Kimmage remained a naif, at least compared to his peers. 'Thierry Claveyrolat used to laugh about it, the notion that I was a doper,' Kimmage recalls of his late former teammate, winner of the 'King of the Mountains' classification in the Tour. Claveyrolat turned on Kimmage when *Rough Ride* was published, soon after the Irishman quit racing. But while Kimmage left the dopers behind and built a career in sports journalism, Claveyrolat was one of those whose life seemed blighted after he retired from racing: there was a car crash, a failing bar business in a claustrophobic Alpine valley and finally a tragic and lonely end. Late one night, after he'd rolled down the shutters and closed up, Claveyrolat blew his brains out in the basement of the bar.

'Cycling's brought you a lot of sadness, hasn't it?' I say to Kimmage.

'No,' says Paul, 'not at all.'

'Are you bitter?' I ask.

'That,' he replies, 'is the perception. For eight years there were degrees of it, yes, until the Festina Affair. Maybe it's an air I give off sometimes, but then after Festina, I had people coming up to me saying, "You were right."

'But why would I be bitter? When I finished cycling in 1990 I walked into a great job on an Irish newspaper that gave me three times the salary I'd earned as a professional bike rider. I had no incentive to write that book, because it was only going to be trouble. It would have been the easiest thing in the world to go back to the Tour each year, say hello to my great pals, and be one of the boys.'

Kimmage says that he felt betrayed when he was racing. 'I thought, either shoot your mouth off now or you can set out to try and sort it out for the next generation. People forget about the number of kids who have died, kids who I rode with who died a year later. If one of their parents had come up to me and said, "You knew about that . . . *You knew – and you said nothing,*" what's my defence? I haven't got a defence.'

Like Walsh, he has a bone to pick with one particular rider. In Kimmage's case, it's David Millar. Kimmage never liked Millar much in the first place and he certainly does not buy into the notion that a self-confessed doper can be reborn clean.

'One strike and you're out,' he says. 'I find it hard to accept that he is now being heralded as a whistle-blower. He didn't blow any whistles, didn't do any favours to cycling. I don't think he even scratched the surface. With the best will in the world, much as I would like to invest some faith in David Millar, I've no reason to. He has just treated me with total disrespect.'

Kimmage is not optimistic for the Tour's future. 'It's just self-perpetuating,' he says, reiterating that the only mistake I've made is of giving people a second chance. He tells me I'm guilty of believing that people can change for the better. 'They only get one chance,' he says.

His scepticism extends to those who readily offered Millar a route back into the sport. This, I am about to learn, includes myself and others such as David Brailsford, the highly successful performance director of the Great Britain cycling team. I waffle about Millar, his contrition and my hopes that, second time around, he is genuine and sincere. But Kimmage barks back: 'No second chances.' I feel mealy-mouthed, wet, overly liberal in his presence. Kimmage inhabits a black-and-white world and for the second time in five minutes, I am envious.

'Brailsford may be a very gifted man, but I did have serious reservations about him embracing Millar. I found his defence of Millar very strange. I understand he was with Millar when he was arrested, which I'm not sure in his position is a healthy thing. But I got a huge kick out of the fact that he had to tell him to put all his toys away with Luigi Cecchini, even before Millar's second coming.'

A 'huge kick'?

He glares at me. 'When I see Millar welcomed back like a hero . . . I mean – I tried to do the sport a service. But he hasn't shat on any of his pals, he's still playing the game, still respecting the *omerta*. And then he comes back and starts lecturing us about what needs to be done . . . How would that not make you bitter?'

Kimmage carries on talking. The tape is running. I'm listening, but I'm also halfway across a bridge, standing in the middle, my old cosy beliefs behind me and the cold world of the hardliners beckoning. I know now that I need to cross, to join them, but it's hard. Kimmage stands watching from the far bank, burning crosses ranged on the hills behind him, calling me.

Then we're back in the café.

'It's quite clear,' he is saying. 'Millar should not have been let back into the sport. He shoulda been banned for life. Until the sport does that, there's no chance. But Millar . . .' he says more softly, and shakes his head. 'Y'know, I watched this guy. He just oozes class and talent, he's beautiful to watch on a bike. The classiest guy I've ever seen on a bike.'

Don't you think I know that, Paul? That's why it hurts . . . of course I know that.

Like Christophe Bassons and Filippo Simeoni, the whistle-blowers who came a decade or so later, the publication of *Rough Ride* sent Paul Kimmage to a lonely place. He had broken the law of silence. He was quickly ostracised, even by old mates such as Claveyrolat. When he went back to the Tour, in July 1990, he says he endured his ex-teammates spitting in his face.

'They reduced me to nothing,' he remembers.

Contrast Kimmage's return to the sport with Millar's and the reason for his anger with the idea of 'David Millar, whistle-blower' comes more clearly into focus. 'They hadn't read the book, but Stephen Roche had talked to *L'Equipe*, saying that I was screwing everybody. That was enough for them. So when I went back, everybody – *everybody* – in the game thought, "Kimmage has fucked us over." It hurt.'

Kimmage tried to leave his bitterness and pain behind and move on. His career as a writer progressed. Then, when he was at the Atlanta Olympics in 1996 and smelled a rat, the experience of *Rough Ride* served him well.

'There was an Irish swimmer who won three gold medals,' he says, referring to Michelle de Bruin. 'Three writers stood up and said this is not right and I was one of them. If I hadn't written *Rough Ride*, I'd have never been able to take that stance. I could have been accused of having double standards, of being a hypocrite. I didn't understand that in 1990, but I certainly appreciated it in 1996.'

Kimmage says there's nobody he admires more in cycling, at any level, than Christophe Bassons. 'I admire him more than Merckx, Hinault, anybody. He is my absolute hero. I don't know him, never met him, but I admire him more than anybody.'

Bassons' stance against the peer pressure of the Festina team won the Irishman's eternal respect. 'I think about what I did and then about what he did. And for him to do it in that era, with Virenque and these boys mocking him across the table, for him to refuse to do what they did . . .'

We shake hands and part, him for the airport, me for a nearby Tube station. Meeting Kimmage again has been a disturbing experience. He paints a bleak picture and offers no resolution, no soft options, no compromises, no get-out clauses, no flim-flam. Our conversation leaves me drained and wanting to drink a lot of red wine.

Later that night, I empty the last of the bottle into my glass. The next morning, my head fogged, I wake up early and pull the curtains open on a grey and empty dawn.

A SONG FROM UNDER THE
FLOORBOARDS

Initially, Filippo Simeoni agreed to be interviewed for this book, but then, weary of two years of recrimination and legal battles, as a direct result of his conflict with Armstrong, he changed his mind. He and his family had had enough trouble, he said. Speaking out had got him nowhere.

He had expected that the fallout from his spat with Armstrong would last one, maybe two seasons. The Italian had thought that he, like those who had doped and been forgiven, would have been accepted back into the fold. But no: the stand-off with Lance still cast a long shadow over his life. For those who cross Armstrong, there is usually no way back.

When he got back home from Paris in July 2004, Filippo Simeoni received a lot of support. The legendary Italian national selector Alfredo Martini sent him a letter telling him, 'It's Armstrong that wants to destroy cycling – not you.' He continued racing, competing in the GP Camaiore, where once again, he came face to face with his chief tormentors. Almost to a man, they ignored him. Only Andrea Peron made an attempt to apologise. Simeoni waved him away.

It was a taste of things to come. Simeoni's initial support faded and Armstrong won the battle for hearts and minds. Filippo spoke to his uncle in Canada, keen to find out how the North American media had handled their confrontation. His anger turned to bitterness when he was told that there had hardly been any coverage, and that what little there was had taken Armstrong's side. At *procycling* we received a flurry of emails, mostly from rabid Lance fans, branding Simeoni a 'whiner, a doper and a loser'. For a while, it all gave him extra motivation. The greatest irony came late that season, when for the first time, on the back of some good results, he was picked for the Italian national team. Most of his teammates barely spoke to him but nonetheless, Simeoni was jubilant to represent his country.

He felt vindicated when the Italian federation later began a disciplinary procedure against Giuseppe Guerini – the same Guerini who subsequently mentored young riders at T-Mobile – over his abuse of Simeoni during the 2004 Tour. Shortly before a hearing could be held, Guerini sent a letter of apology and any action against him was dropped. Most of the others barely felt any ill-effects, however; at the end of 2004 'Pippo' Pozzato, still seen by many as the great hope of Italian cycling, was elected head of the Italian riders' association. Predictably, Simeoni was appalled.

Two procedures pitting Simeoni against Armstrong looked possible, the first for intimidating a witness – *in a bicycle race?* – the second, more sustainable, for defamation. The painfully slow progress of the Italian legal system had ensured that the trial against Michele Ferrari was still ongoing in July 2004. When the Italian judiciary saw what had happened at the Tour between Simeoni and Armstrong, it started paying close attention. Simeoni had been a witness in that trial and Armstrong, so Simeoni claimed, had threatened him: hence the possibility of an intimidation charge.

The defamation suit arose from the interview Armstrong had given to *Le Monde*, in which he had denounced Simeoni as a *'menteur absolu'* – an absolute liar. Belatedly, Simeoni and his lawyer decided to act. Yet, for a combination of reasons – bad timing, Simeoni's own recalcitrance, and the labyrinthian complexities of the Italian judicial system and cycling scene – neither case went to court. Simeoni, despairing, believed it had all been for nothing.

He was wrong. His actions had accelerated change, even if

that change would come too late, much too late, to salvage his own career.

Simeoni started 2006 in a positive frame of mind, but then in the spring he battened down the hatches when he found himself increasingly isolated. His campaigning stance against doping had not endeared him to the Italian sports media.

Simeoni had never pretended to be a saint. He had admitted to doping himself, which he testified to following his consultations with Michele Ferrari. But, depicted as a chest-beating evangelist by the press, he found the criticism hard to take. *Who does he think he is?* they wrote. *Just an ex-doper with a guilty conscience who confessed under the pressure of police investigation.* Those criticisms may well have influenced his decision to withdraw, but it's more likely that it was the refusal of cycling's elite teams in the ProTour to offer him a contract that finally shut Simeoni up.

Vincenzo Santoni, Simeoni's manager in 2006 at the Naturino team, had told the Italian that he would release him from the final year of his contract, if a ProTour team was willing to take him. But in a paranoid sport, Simeoni divided loyalties. Despite his abilities as an athlete and despite discreet support from other high-profile riders, Simeoni was not in demand. In desperation, at the end of 2006, he wrote a letter to every ProTour team saying that he was still keen to race at the very highest level. None responded.

Fellow Italian pro Gilberto Simoni asked around at several teams, including his own, Saunier Duval, on Filippo's behalf. Ironically, Simoni's sponsor also had another reformed ex-doper, David Millar, on their books. But Millar was different. And, after his two-year ban, he had been accepted back into the peloton.

For his part, Gilberto Simoni had always been complimentary about Filippo, believing he'd make a 'brilliant *domestique*' for a grand-tour specialist. But neither the words of a former Giro d'Italia champion and Tour de France stage winner, nor the growing acceptance that doping was crippling the sport, were enough. David Millar may have experienced a kind of redemption, but Simeoni, *persona non grata*, remained exiled by the elite.

According to his close friends, Filippo has a figure in his head of how much it has all cost him – the row with Armstrong, the things he's said about doping. Simeoni believes it all adds up to hundreds of thousands of euros, small beer to affluent superstars like Riis and Armstrong, but a fortune to a *domestique*.

When he quits racing, Filippo Simeoni plans to devote himself to running the café he owns with his brother, in Sezze, Tuscany. His final seasons will help to make up for the lost income and the humiliation he has endured since he broke the *omerta*.

Part Three
Doing the Right Thing

'Those who cannot remember the past are condemned to repeat it.'

George Santayana

BLAME IT ON THE BADGER

When it was announced that the 1994 Tour de France would visit England, I was beside myself with excitement. On a pigeon-grey morning in Trafalgar Square, when Bernard Hinault was scheduled for a photocall to publicise the Tour's visit, I skipped work and made a pilgrimage to see the legendary Badger, 'Le Blaireau' – so called because cornered badgers always come out fighting, although having never personally baited a French badger I can't verify this – in the flesh.

For a long time, I endured an overpowering sense of sadness and melancholia over Hinault's premature retirement at just thirty-two, when a sixth Tour win would surely have been possible. I felt deprived, peeved even. In the fantasy Tour in my head, in which Eddy Merckx took on Fausto Coppi, and Greg LeMond struggled to contain Charly Gaul, no other rider compared to him. I missed his narcissistic macho posturing, his arrogant taunting of his rivals, his mocking of their masculine inadequacies, as he strutted around like some demented porn star. Certainly, I hadn't suffered this morbid state of depression when, for example, the big-nosed, balding Italian, Massimo Ghirotto, hung up his racing wheels.

But Hinault's growling good looks, his Breton granite physique, his tendency to six o'clock shadow, his love of Ray-Ban Aviators and his D'Artagnan smile, allied to his pugilistic bloody-mindedness, had all made him so appealing. In the bland age of monosyllabic Miguel Indurain and 'Swiss Tony' Rominger, his flamboyant and outspoken personality was sorely missed.

The robotic anonymity of the new champions of the early 1990s made them the anti-Hinault. The Badger was the kind of reckless Frenchman who relished risk, a have-a-go hero who'd roar up to your back bumper at the wheel of a soft-top Peugeot, gesticulating wildly and cursing, flashing his lights and hooting, before shooting you a devil-may-care grin and swerving past on a blind hairpin, narrowly missing a Belgian camper van as he did so.

Yes, at times he could be a bit of a twat.

No pilgrimage to meet the Breton would have been complete without a copy of his absurdly bombastic biography, *Memories of the Peloton*, as Napoleonic and self-aggrandising a text as in any French oeuvre. Clutching the hardback in my sweaty paw as I emerged from the Northern Line, I nervously rehearsed a few lines of French with which to charm Saint Bernard. Perhaps we would fall into conversation, and laugh and joke; then, showing his trademark impetuosity, he would tear up his schedule, wave his minders away and suggest we head off for lunch, somewhere discreet and intimate, up the road in Soho.

But then they always warn you about meeting your heroes, don't they?

I spotted the familiar figure adrift among a sea of Japanese tourists, loitering under Nelson's Column, clad in a shiny green suit that must have lit up like a Christmas tree when he took it off at night. Unflatteringly, it also revealed the beginnings of a paunch, and was so ill-fitting that it displayed an alarming length of white towelling sock above his pig-nosed shoes.

Was this the athletic colossus whose duel with LeMond had fired my dreams, who had conquered Galibier, Tourmalet, Ventoux, who had ridden alone through the blizzard-swept Belgian Ardennes to win Liège-Bastogne-Liège, crossing the finish line with frozen hands and icicles dangling from his bike frame (if not his nose)? Was this the proud man of the soil who had played such sophisticated mind games with LeMond that the American had been reduced to a nervous wreck, the same man who had ridden with such carefree panache that all France had flocked to lionise him?

No – this was a middle-aged French farmer in a bad suit on an away day.

I took a deep breath and walked up to him. '*Bonjour, Monsieur Hinault,*' I said. '*Comment ça va?*'

He glanced at me, smiled a tight smile and continued talking to a similarly green-suited colleague from the Tour organisation about lunch or taxis or how much longer he had to stand here in this draughty London square.

There was a pause. What should I say? How could I break the ice? 'So did you laugh when Greg got mistaken for a turkey?' might have raised a quizzical eyebrow, but would also perhaps have struck the wrong note.

So I settled for '*U-un signature, s'il vous plaît . . .*' and I thrust the book at him. He scribbled something and pushed it back into my hand, before turning on his heel and striding off towards a waiting taxi. Another sea of tourists came between us and then he was gone. I should have known. Nobody puts The Badger in a corner.

I stood there clutching the signed book amid the pigeons and the tourists. The sense of anticlimax left me swooning. Heroes – *hah*! What are they good for?

In July 2007, thirteen years after my brief encounter with Hinault, the Tour returned to London and south-east England. This time it arrived against the backdrop of Ken Livingstone's two-wheeled Utopia, of London as Olympus, a city of sporting excellence and endeavour, a city where cabbies and bus drivers looked on admiringly as you pedalled past pavement cafés through perpetually sunlit streets, rather than spitting vitriol and abuse as you got in their way when a rutted cycle lane suddenly dropped into a rainwater-filled crater deeper than the Grand Canyon.

This time the Tour de France was welcomed with open arms to the heart of the capital, with one of the most beautiful prologue routes, slaloming through Whitehall, St James's, Hyde Park and the Mall. This time the Tour was the answer, to obesity, slothfulness, congestion, xenophobia and environmental catastrophe. The bicycle remained simple, beautiful and clean, even as the Tour – the bloody Tour – just kept on getting dirtier.

SHOOTING THE MESSENGER

'Cycling,' said Dick Pound, the no-nonsense agent provocateur and former head of the World Anti-Doping Agency (WADA), 'is in the toilet.'

In his time as WADA's figurehead, this mild-mannered, carefully spoken man, with a clipped Canadian accent, became the principal hate object for dopers all around the world. I always had the impression that he rather enjoyed that status. His reputation was definitively forged by his involvement in the Salt Lake City Olympic corruption investigation. He built his career in what he described as 'sports administration' after a youth spent competing as an Olympic and Commonwealth swimmer.

In essence, WADA's role is principally that of a campaigning watchdog. It monitors the success of anti-doping measures in sport, suggests improvements and establishes educational programmes so that athletes are better informed. But Pound, as president of WADA, took it a step further and added 'ruffling feathers' to his job description.

He did this remarkably effectively in cycling, one of the sports that he considers most damaged by doping. Among those he greatly pissed off during his tenure of the WADA presidency were former president of the UCI, Hein Verbruggen, Lance Armstrong and Floyd Landis. Pound seemed tickled by the thought of many of cycling's most high-profile figures loathing – and fearing – him.

Among professional athletes, Pound was as welcome as Ebenezer Scrooge on Christmas morning. A lot of sports fans felt the same way. Pound's remit, after all, was to destroy their illusions. Visit the forum or message boards of almost any sports website and there will be a series of rants about Dick Pound and his attitude problem, telling him to leave a star athlete alone. Pound always accepted that this came with the territory.

'The nature of the job is to upset the established order which has allowed doping to proliferate. I'm quite happy to be known by the enemies I make. In fact, if you haven't made enemies, I'd say you're not doing the job. One of the roles is to try and raise the level of the public's understanding that there really is a problem out there.'

WADA has become increasingly influential, since it was created in 1999, as a direct response to the Festina drug scandal. 'The groundwork for WADA was laid as early as August 1998, after the Festina Affair,' Pound explained. 'We got together and I said nobody believes anybody any more. They don't believe that cycling – or any international federation – will police its own sport properly. They don't believe national authorities will look after their own athletes properly and they don't believe in the IOC any more. So we needed an independent agency, which led to the creation of WADA. In the process of all that, I was asked to run it, but I didn't know anything about doping, and I'd damn near killed myself doing the Salt Lake City investigations – I didn't want to do it.'

Pound says that his appointment as head of WADA was presented to him as a fait accompli. He knew that after the Salt Lake City investigation, he was hardly a popular choice.

'I think people understood that I could organise things and that I had no interest in covering up doping. They may not have expected the kind of progress we've made over the last few years. I'm sure if some of the international federations had realised how far we'd get, then they would have been much more concerned about my involvement.'

He soon came into conflict with cycling's hierarchy. 'I can remember, long before I was involved in anti-doping, discussing cycling's ethical problems with Hein Verbruggen, when he was president of the UCI, before the Festina Affair. I was saying, "Hein, you have got a real problem in your sport and you don't seem able to deal with it." He said, "Well, listen – if people don't mind the Tour de France at twenty-five kilometres per hour, the riders don't have to prepare – but if they want it at forty-two kilometres per hour, then I'm sorry, the riders can't do it without preparation," as he called it.' Verbruggen has dismissed Pound's claims as 'nonsense' and denies that Pound ever spoke to him about a specific problem in cycling.

Pound never felt confident that Verbruggen was prepared to 'rock the boat'. 'Look at the multimillion-dollar headquarters that the UCI have in Aigle in Switzerland,' he said. 'That doesn't come from amateur track cycling.'

Pound believed that Verbruggen's skills were not right for the problems the UCI faced. 'I don't know what the UCI's marketing objectives were, although I think that you could probably do some research and find that Verbruggen's forte as a professional was in marketing.'

That's right, I said. His background was in milk and Mars bars.

'There's no possible or credible way that cycling can say, "We don't have a problem." And football has actually said, "There's nothing on the WADA list that would help any footballer." When you get leaders in sport saying things as outrageous as that, then they have to be confronted.'

Pound didn't give anybody an easy time. He argued that the media have been compromised by their cosy relationships. 'The media – and maybe I'm generalising here, because obviously there are journalists who want to get at these things – have been *very* compliant, getting the press releases and going to the press conferences, having a glass of wine, some food and listening to stuff that's churned out by people who are paid a lot of money to pretend there's no problem.'

Doping, he said, is not one of the 'shades of grey'. 'This is cheating and for the most part it's organised cheating. You have to confront it. Maybe people thought that I would be . . .

more European than I am and try and do it quietly behind the scenes, with handshakes and winks and things like that. But I don't think that's what you do to draw attention to a problem of this nature. It is ethically wrong, fraudulent and causes misery for athletes and their families. Here are the rules: we're not going to use certain drugs and doping methods. It's as simple as that.'

In March 2005, a few years after my initial request, Hein Verbruggen, at the time still president of the UCI, finally agreed to a face-to-face interview.

In the dining room of the Long Beach Sheraton, I walked over to his breakfast table. He put his coffee cup down and stood up. We shook hands.

'How are you, Mr Verbruggen?' I said.

There was a pause.

'You write too much about doping,' he told me.

Doping already? Here we go, I thought.

I didn't expect to get on with Hein Verbruggen.

In 1998 he had written to *The Times*, and demanded an apology – rather pompously adding 'on behalf of Jean-Marie Leblanc', the Tour de France's director – for a piece I had written on the Festina Affair. He'd also put the phone down on me on more than one occasion during the *procycling* years, once memorably bellowing into his mobile from some distant corner of Switzerland, 'Mr Whittle, I am *sick of you* and your *bullshit* magazine.'

Yet, sipping a Starbucks latte in a Californian hotel lounge overlooking the Pacific, he was all charm, largesse and dry wit. Thoughtful and articulate, he gave me two hours of his time. I warmed to him. Let's make a fresh start, I thought. Let bygones be bygones.

I had planned to keep the doping questions for later on, but he was straight into it, talking of corruption, race fixing and EPO within five minutes of sitting down. He joshed with me about what he perceived as the British obsession with honour and fair play and suddenly I remembered that, yes, of course – Hein's a salesman, Hein's a liberaliser and Hein's from Holland.

As we talked, the cultural differences between us came into sharper focus. Hein was weary of the infighting. He wants us Europeans to get along. We should stop carping and understand that things in cycling are a damn sight better than they were. We should chill, relax.

It was only a few months since David Millar's downfall, and despite the fact that Millar admitted doping to win the UCI's own World Time Trial title, Verbruggen showed bonhomie and forgiveness. 'How is David Millar, by the way?' he asked. 'Give him my warm regards if you see him.'

Unlike his many critics, Verbruggen believes he dragged cycling from the darkness into the modern ages. He illustrated this by telling me, unprompted, about the mess he inherited when he became UCI president in the mid 1980s. 'It was an era when doping flourished – although I am not saying that everybody was doped – I'd be the last to say that. But there were insufficient controls, not enough regulations or professionalism. A group of people within the sport saw that things couldn't go on like that, organisers like Jean-Marie Leblanc, team managers like Roger Legeay and others within the UCI. I'd say that we have excellent professionals within the UCI now. We have a rulebook, and we have much better controls for doping.'

So this then – the post-Festina, pre-Puerto era, the eight years sandwiched between the two biggest scandals in cycling's history, – was Hein Verbruggen's new dawn.

Dick Pound believes that cycling's 'deep, deep problem' still exists. 'I don't think the problem has gone away, I think it's got worse.'

The root of it all, he says, is money. Doping, he says, is big business. 'These are not just little tablets you take out of a supplement bottle. The riders are paying tens of thousands of euros a year for medical treatment and preparation.'

Cycling's high profile, particularly in Europe, means that doping scandals, like Festina and Puerto, have been big news, but, he adds, 'it's not the only sport with a doping problem.'

He reels off the major scandals of the past ten years and concludes that there have been so many busts, particularly in the Tour, that it's akin to having the entire field in the Olympic final of the 100 metres disqualified.

'A few years ago, the public watching the Tour might have said, "I wonder if any of them are using drugs," and now they say, "I wonder if any of them are *not* using drugs." That's the price you pay, the price that all sports pay, for letting things get out of hand.'

Dick Pound wanted cycling to step up to the plate, to take responsibility. 'We gave them suggestions on their testing programme, which we thought was very ineffective and designed "around" the problem, rather than to catch dopers. Up until recently,' Pound argued, 'the fight against doping has been pretty limited. If you didn't find traces of a substance in an athlete's system, then there was no doping. Yet all the people in the entourages were going unchecked and unsanctioned. Now, with public authorities able to go in and seize evidence and question witnesses, it gives us a much broader ability to get the enablers, suppliers and the medical practitioners who are assisting in all this. It gives us a much more vigorous arsenal of weapons.'

Sounds great, I say, this arsenal of weapons – police raids, secret surveillance, informers, DNA testing and so on – but what happened to athletes not doping themselves because it is wrong? What happened to the ideals of fair play, honour, respect for your rival – all the things that lift sport out of the maelstrom of everyday life and give it real meaning?

'Yep,' says Dick Pound. 'I know. I agree entirely. There are sociopaths out there. That's why we have a police force. That's why we have security checks at airports. That's an unfortunate fact of life. We're now paying the price for the sports authorities letting this get out of control and closing their eyes to it.'

Hein Verbruggen and Dick Pound have history. They used to be friends, but are not any more. They have both been key members of the International Olympic Committee's hierarchy. Now, because of the confrontational positions they took over doping, they are virtually estranged.

'I don't care about Mr Pound because he is not objective,' said Verbruggen. 'I don't want to see him any more. He was a good friend of mine but he's not now. WADA should be on the federation's side but many federations have a problem with him. But we can't solve the problem of doping without working with governments and that's what WADA do.

'Pound's the sheriff who shoots everything that moves. WADA should be above all that and he should establish proof before he speaks. Athletes have the right to defend themselves – even if it's with the cheapest excuse.'

Maybe it's because of Verbruggen's professional background in marketing that Pound irritates him so much. He sees himself as a unifier. He doesn't want confrontation, but a quiet revolution at his own pace, that styles cycling on other successful sports franchises.

'Look at basketball in the USA. Look at the Champions League in European soccer – I don't want to compare cycling with those sports, only the system. If you work together, you get much more,' he enthused. 'It's about making the cake bigger – you combine forces and it makes you stronger.'

That may explain why, by his own admission, he embraced the boom in road cycling among Americans. It may also explain his determination to defend his tainted creation, the ProTour, the pan-European calendar of elite races that was intended to showcase the top teams and riders, bringing with it a torrent of franchise and TV revenues – the same ProTour that didn't want an athlete like Filippo Simeoni muddying its waters.

'I am European, so I think in a European way. But I am not too old to learn and take some good things from other cultures. In the States, maybe they talk a bit too much about money, but you can even learn from that.'

Verbruggen's fervour for the American way may also have been coloured by the legend of Lance. 'What the Tour has done for France is incredible. If you put a value on that, it would be worth billions of euros. But the TV companies are there to cover the race, not the countryside. They're there to cover the riders.'

The importance of Lance Armstrong to the growth in popularity of the Tour de France has been huge. For once, he said, the old adage about no single rider being greater than the Tour is wrong. By the end of his career, Armstrong, Verbruggen believed, was bigger than the race that had made him. This, Verbruggen said, was because Armstrong had 'a lot of charisma, a very strong personality'.

But the Dutchman's and the Texan's mutually beneficial friendship made some uneasy. Verbruggen always waved away suggestions of a 'special' relationship, but it has been acknowledged by both men that the UCI received unspecified financial donations from Armstrong.

'He gave money for research against doping, to discover new anti-doping methods,' Verbruggen revealed. 'He gave money from his private funds, cash. He didn't want this to be known but he did it.'

In a television interview on Eurosport, Armstrong later confirmed that he had given 'a fair amount' to the UCI. 'It wasn't a small amount of money,' he said. But exactly how much was donated, nobody knows. Some, like Germany's former UCI committee member Sylvia Schenk, have speculated that it might have been up to $500,000.

'We had no official information on the donation and, as a member of the UCI board, I wanted to know about it,' Schenk said at the offices of her law firm in Frankfurt. 'I asked how much was paid, when it was paid, but I never got any information. And as far as I know, it is still not clear exactly how much money was donated by Lance Armstrong and what it was used for. I don't understand why the UCI won't say how much it was and when it was paid.'

Schenk's inquisitive nature didn't endear her to the UCI president. She says that Verbruggen stopped talking to her in May 2004. 'I was still a member of the UCI board, but he wasn't talking to me. Whatever I suggested, regarding for example the ProTour, I was ignored. That was the way they dealt with me for years.' Schenk was 'very surprised' by Armstrong's donation. 'It's not what athletes usually do. It's unusual to hear about it so much later, six months, or a year later, via the media. It already seemed to be a secret. I don't know why. So, of course there are doubts now.'

Even Armstrong himself acknowledged that he preferred the details of his donation to remain secret. 'It is not my modus operandi to advertise what I do,' he said. 'If I've given money to the UCI to combat doping, step up controls and to fund research, it is not my job to issue a press release. That's a secret thing, because it's the right thing to do. I am not the type of person who likes to get up and say in the newspaper, "Our sport is dirty, everyone is cheating." There are other avenues to combat doping, versus trashing the sport and its players, its sponsors and spectators.'

Whatever Schenk's concerns, Verbruggen remains a big Lance fan. He told me the story of an award that had been given to Armstrong in France. 'You know, of course, that two journalists had written a book about him published in France, yet despite that, the French gave him this prize. It's significant that this jury was not influenced by gossip.

'If you saw what Lance has to go through! I think they controlled him maybe five or six times last Christmas. That's five or six times – out of competition – at seven o'clock in the morning, at his house.'

★   ★   ★

Drug testing in cycling has always been reactive, rather than proactive. It took the death of Tom Simpson on Mont Ventoux during the 1967 Tour for the governing bodies, under public pressure, to move towards the introduction of doping controls. Until that time, doping had been swept under the carpet, even though riders such as Jacques Anquetil, who won five Tours, had openly acknowledged the widespread use of drugs such as amphetamines.

'You'd have to be an imbecile or a hypocrite to imagine that a professional cyclist who rides 235 days a year can hold himself together without stimulants,' the Frenchman said.

Simpson's death was a wake-up call. The following year's race in July 1968 was christened the 'Tour de Sante'. But the peloton was hardly wholehearted in its support: a rider's strike greeted the first doping controls. In truth, they have been complaining about them ever since. Even in 2007, in the aftermath of Operacíon Puerto and the disgrace of Floyd Landis, the notion of DNA profiling produced a knee-jerk reaction from many top professionals. Showing the public relations skills that had characterised the sport for more than a decade, leading riders claimed indignantly that such a move aligned them with murderers and rapists, and would infringe their human rights.

The introduction of the the fifty per cent haematocrit controls in 1997 came only after it became apparent that EPO use had reached epidemic levels during the mid 1990s. To Hein Verbruggen, this was a timely and radical intervention, rather than a Band-Aid on a haemorrhage.

'We started doing it before the Festina Affair happened. Now, everybody is realising what we have done. What our athletes have to comply with now in terms of anti-doping is outstanding; but a big problem you always have with doping is that the riders are suspicious of each other. "What has he got that I haven't? Don't I have to do the same as him?"'

But the introduction of the fifty per cent haematocrit 'health check' also heralded the downfall of riders such as Marco Pantani.

The consequences for him, both as an athlete and a human being, were catastrophic. Even Verbruggen can't argue with this assessment.

'It's true. He was never the same again. I was there that day. And it was a terrible day. I liked the guy, he was extremely popular. But the whole system for those controls was set up with the teams and the riders. The riders had all signed and agreed. Pantani was one of them, the most popular one.'

Verbruggen says that he regrets that a foolproof EPO test had not been introduced sooner. 'We'd been trying since 1993. During that year's World Championships Francesco Conconi told me that they were very close to a validated test. That year was when we started to have concerns that EPO was in the peloton. After that we waited and waited, until in 1996, when I again met with Conconi at the Olympic Games in Atlanta. People think he was in the UCI's anti-doping commission but that's wrong. He was in our medical commission and that commission had a responsibility for cardiology, trauma, nutrition and training methods. He was developing the test, together with members of the IOC medical commission.'

But did the UCI entrust the study of haematocrit controls to the right man? Among Conconi's protégés, during his time teaching medicine in Italian universities and working with athletes in the 1980s, were Michele Ferrari and Luigi Cecchini, yet Verbruggen fails to see any conflict in Conconi's involvement with the development of a desperately needed EPO test.

Instead, he maintains, the battle to introduce a haematocrit test and control the abuse of EPO, was won by Conconi. 'Conconi deserves the recognition for this. He persuaded top riders to accept the haematocrit controls. On 24 January, 1997, we got all the teams and doctors together and we decided on haematocrit controls and at the same time on a medical control system. Because the EPO test still wasn't ready.'

And the first rider to be caught, I am thinking, was Erwann Mentheour − a client of Michele Ferrari.

OK, I said, but wasn't the test intrinsically unfair? We may suspect, but will never know, definitively, if Pantani had EPO in his system on the day he failed the test, yet his life took a tragic turn because of that uncertainty.

'Nobody wanted to wait. It was a real problem in the peloton. And some of the team leaders I talked to said, "The riders don't want to use the stuff but they keep losing races." At the time, I think we did what we could.'

But the haematocrit test was a smokescreen. It did virtually nothing to prevent or discourage doping. Many riders carried on using EPO. And given the opinions of many haematologists, the variations in natural levels and the effect of intense competition and fatigue on red blood cells, why establish the level at fifty per cent based on tests conducted halfway through a mountainous stage race?

Cue more agitation on the other side of the Sheraton's polished coffee table.

'I saw an interview with Giorgio Squinzi' – the Italian ceramics magnate who sponsored the Mapei team – 'he never liked the UCI very much and I didn't like him. He said that having a haematocrit level set at fifty per cent was the same as telling people that they could steal up to $1,000! That is *so* bloody stupid,' raged Verbruggen, 'and there are still people who are willing to print this nonsense.'

I'm sorry – but 'bloody stupid'?

Bloody stupid that a wonder drug that its users say can improve performance by up to twenty per cent was tacitly legalised?

Bloody stupid, when all research points out that haematocrit varies so greatly between individuals that it is almost impossible to agree a standard, particularly one of fifty per cent?

Bloody stupid, when Marco Pantani ended his life face down in a cheap hotel room, his career and reputation ruined – by a UCI 'health check'?

FROM A WHISPER TO A SCREAM

When Lance Armstrong retired from racing, the Tour de France fell apart.

Without the Texan bossing the European scene, the house of cards finally collapsed. The despair and paranoia that had characterised the 1998 Tour and the Festina Affair flooded back into the sport. It was as if the Lance years of limitless wealth and unquestioned glory had all been a mirage, a dream. The whispers of widespread doping, suppressed between 1999 and 2005, as Armstrong's became the dominant voice in the sport, became a scream.

Armstrong had finally quit centre stage in July 2005, standing alongside Jan Ullrich and Ivan Basso on the Paris podium, chastising the non-believers.

'To the people who don't believe in cycling,' he said, 'the cynics and the sceptics, I'm sorry you don't believe in miracles, but this is a hell of a race. You should believe in these athletes, and you should believe in these people.'

These turned out to be empty words. Twenty-four hours before the start of the following year's Tour in Strasbourg, Basso and Ullrich were kicked off the race.

Planted at the easternmost point of a vast plain that stretches from Champagne to the German border, Strasbourg, a city infamous for its bitter winters and broiling summers, welcomed the opening weekend of the first Tour of the post-Armstrong era.

Strasbourg is a genteel and conservative city of bike lanes and pedestrianisation, trams and cobbled squares, a towering cathedral at its heart. There is no litter or graffiti. In July 2006, as the World Cup neared its climax and Ullrich and Basso scuttled home in disgrace, sporadic football chants broke out, but that came only as the crowds spilled out from the bars around the cathedral, waving tricolour flags and singing the praises of Zinedine Zidane. For an hour or two, the city seemed almost rowdy, but soon after midnight, shutters were pulled closed and the streets were empty again.

If the World Cup and France's unexpected success had fuelled a sense of celebration, the Grand Depart of the 2006 Tour quickly became a poorly attended wake. Armstrong's retirement had left the door open for either of his old rivals to succeed him. Basso was fresh from a runaway win in the Giro d'Italia and Ullrich had added another Tour of Switzerland victory to his name.

But twenty-four hours before the race started, as the Operacíon Puerto doping investigation in Spain became the biggest scandal since the Festina Affair, both of them found themselves wide-eyed, frozen out, blinking in the TV lights and flashguns as their careers caved in.

Even after everything that has happened in cycling since the Festina Affair, it still doesn't pay to speak out against doping. Just ask Ivan Basso. Confronted by the Italian Olympic Committee (CONI) over his connections to Eufemiano Fuentes and his blood banks, Basso confessed only to contemplating doping, rather than the act itself. The Italian remained loyal to the half-truths of the *omerta*, and was inscrutable, evasive, discreet.

When, his 2006 racing season torn in half by Operacíon Puerto, he finally confessed, not to doping, you understand, but instead to just thinking about it, he shrugged his shoulders, as if he was a Rimini nightclubber pondering the price of a tab. His half-hearted admission was greeted with derision, yet Ivan still didn't get it. Even months later, as he continued to train and plan his comeback, he was baffled by the contempt that had greeted his sly admission of a moment of weakness.

Basso had begun 2006, training in Italy, as CSC's star rider and Armstrong's heir apparent. At the team's January get-together, in the Hotel Caesar in Tuscany, he had been accorded star status. Bjarne Riis had made Basso into a contender. With his help, he had lost his hesitancy and come out of his shell. At the team's midwinter 'boot camps', Ivan had learned to make fear his friend. He had forced himself to overcome his nerves, jumping off cliff tops into a dark and icy sea, while Bjarne looked on, grinning.

The alliance with Riis had fast-tracked Basso's progress. He was brimming with confidence and ambition. His test results on Monte Serra's steep climb at the start of 2006 were said to be fifty seconds better than a year earlier. By any standards, he had made phenomenal progress.

Riis wanted Basso to fill the vacuum at the top of the sport; there would be no more living in the shadow of Lance. Even when locked in rivalry with Armstrong during the Tour, Basso had remained in the American's thrall, calling him during the race to offer his 'help'. Riis had not approved of the friendship, established when Lance tried to help the Italian find the best possible care for his mother Nives, at that time seriously ill with cancer. It irritated Riis, who had spent so long in the shadow of the Armstrong-Bruyneel partnership.

Halfway through the 2005 Tour I asked Riis if Basso – like Ullrich – was suffering from an 'Armstrong complex'.

'Isn't everybody?' he replied enigmatically, with that icy, distant smile.

With Armstrong retired, Ivan had hoped to ease himself into the king's vacant chair. He adopted the Texan's intimidatory style, gently admonishing young journalists who asked silly questions about doping. Ivan, like Armstrong, didn't like insinuations about doping, nor did he like doping whistle-blowers. In particular, he didn't like compatriot Filippo Simeoni, who he dismissesd as a '*testa di cazzo*' – a dickhead.

He also found himself struggling with his loyalties. Bruyneel and Armstrong had courted Basso, lining him up as the successor to the US Postal-Discovery Channel dynasty. But the Italian opted to stay with Riis and CSC. Now, he would become a 'capo', a don. He planned to win the Giro d'Italia and the Tour in the same season, just like Marco Pantani had done in 1998.

Success would ensure legendary status – perhaps he might even replace the late lamented Pantani in the *tifosi*'s affections. Victory in the Tour de France would make the transition complete. Armstrong and Bruyneel, meanwhile, would be left to kick a few cats, as the rider who slipped through their fingers became the hottest property in the sport.

As darkness fell outside the hotel, and a wintry sun dropped into the Tuscan horizon, I waited in the bar to talk to the rider touted as cycling's next dominant champion. Team press officer Brian Nygaard led me down the hotel corridors to Ivan's room. We stood in the doorway as the Italian held court from his massage table.

Carlos Sastre, his teammate, was also there, outlining a problem he had with his racing shoes. As the unassuming Sastre looked on, Basso gave instructions to CSC staff. Finally, after a wave of his hand, the room cleared and Basso beckoned me to his side.

'*Ciao Ivan, come stai?*' I said, exhausting my Italian in a single sentence. We had met before, when he was a virtual unknown. Like now, that was also a rushed encounter. Nonetheless he outlined his grand plan. The Giro was his priority, he said; riding the Giro and Tour would not be too hard, he could win both; he hadn't spoken to Lance much because Lance, you see, was always so busy and yes, he and Bjarne had a *very* close working relationship.

'I have a stronger personality now,' Basso said. 'Bjarne likes to hear what I think and doesn't just tell me to do this or that. He's open-minded.'

Three months later, Basso won the Giro d'Italia with ease and arrogance. It brought him the affection of the *tifosi*. They loved him, although not in the same unconditional way that they had loved Pantani. But like Pantani in 1998, the extent and ease of Basso's dominance, the new-found swagger that he seemed to relish, was resented by some of his rivals.

Then, just days before the race ended, it all began.

As Ivan Basso neared victory in Milan, the rumours about his Spanish connections gathered pace. There was a flurry of doping allegations emerging in Madrid, centred on Manolo Saiz, *directeur* of the Liberty Seguros team, but which also seemed to connect Basso to sports doctor Eufemiano Fuentes. There were arrests, blood bags, CCTV footage, lists and codenames. Operacíon Puerto was about to devastate European cycling.

Basso denied any involvement, as did Jan Ullrich, also riding the Giro and also, according to the Spanish media, implicated in the affair. This, it turned out, was the calm before the storm. The Madrid raids, just as the 2006 Giro d'Italia reached its climax, kicked away a cornerstone of the cycling establishment and sparked a frenzy of allegations. Saiz was a key figure both in Spain and within cycling as a whole, influential in the modernisation of the sport. He had managed a long line of major stars. He had also walked out on the 1998 Tour, in protest at the police raids during the Festina Affair.

Saiz's arrest was the watershed moment in an investigation that had begun earlier in 2006, with the installation of hidden cameras at two locations in central Madrid. First, the Guardia Civil installed surveillance equipment in a laboratory used by haematologist, Jose Luis Merino Batres. Then, officers from the Spanish UCO investigative unit moved to a nearby address, at Calle Alonso Cano, where an apartment rented by Eufemiano Fuentes became the focal point of the police operation. When in late May they raided both addresses, they found over two hundred bags of blood, steroids, growth hormone and, of course, the ubiquitous EPO.

The police arrested Saiz after he met both Fuentes and Batres in a Madrid café. He had with him a suitcase containing a large amount of cash. Fuentes in turn arrived with a cold bag. There was a discreet exchange between them, which the police video-taped. When Saiz was stopped after leaving the meeting, a search of the bag revealed coded bags of blood and other products, all of which, so the police claimed, were the paraphernalia of doping.

By the time the Tour set up camp in Strasbourg, the connections between Fuentes and certain riders appeared irrefutable. In an unprecedented display of unity, it was the ProTour teams themselves, forced into action by their own ethical code which stated that riders implicated in police investigations should be suspended, that agreed to eject those involved. Faced with damning allegations against Ullrich and Basso, neither T-Mobile nor CSC had much choice.

In total, nine riders were sent home from the Tour, even before it began. Johan Bruyneel, *directeur* of the Discovery Channel team, which was at that time unaffected by the Puerto investigation, was among the most voluble supporters of a hard-line stance.

For Basso and Ullrich, Strasbourg was a catastrophe. In the aftermath of their expulsion, both of them were implored to take DNA tests, but they refused. Basso's sly smile remained fixed on his face when he appeared at the back of the Holiday Inn and fought his way through the media before climbing into a car and speeding away. Ullrich stood glassy-eyed in front of the camera crews, and gave a half-hearted defence of his reputation, reiterating that he was innocent. Then he too was gone, installing American Floyd Landis of the Phonak team, formerly teammate to Lance Armstrong, as the new race favourite.

After Basso left, Riis, with CSC press officer Brian Nygaard by his side, appeared before the media, in an attempt to defend his team leader and, by proxy, himself. They were jostled and hemmed in by camera crews, photographers and journalists as they made their way into the Strasbourg media centre.

Riis, perhaps through his naivety, or perhaps through arrogance, seemed unperturbed by the mayhem around him. Then I realised why. 'You must be getting used to this, Bjarne . . .' I thought, remembering the chaos of the Festina Affair.

Riis confirmed that the decision to take Basso out of CSC's Tour team had been his, but he was vague about Basso's dealings with Fuentes. Suddenly, it seemed that Bjarne and Basso were not so close after all. 'It's impossible to watch somebody twenty-four hours a day,' he shrugged as he struggled to distance himself from his team leader in a rambling and self-justifying monologue, in which he said a lot, but clarified little.

Back in Spain, Operacíon Puerto threatened to be an earthquake. In the 500-page police report, a list of 200-odd leading athletes were connected to Fuentes and his activities. Other professional sports – tennis, football, athletics – were rumoured to be involved. The UCI's recently elected president, Pat McQuaid, seemed deeply confused even as he fuelled that notion, saying that 'footballers, tennis players and athletes were on the list'. His comments were recorded on tape, yet he almost immediately retracted them, only to reassert them at the World Championships in Salzburg three months later.

Rafael Nadal, playing at Wimbledon, pre-empted any negative publicity by denying rumours of an allegation connecting him to Fuentes. At the World Cup, FIFA laughed off the suggestion that some of those still playing in the competition might have been among Fuentes' clients. Doping was apparently only cycling's problem.

It seemed certain that the net would tighten and that heads would roll. But soon after the 2006 Tour ended, the problems with furthering the investigation began. The codes labelling each bag of blood and in Fuentes' records had to be matched to individual riders. Who, for example, was 'Birillo'? Who was 'amigo di Birillo'? The Spanish media, supported by the claims of those in Italy and elsewhere who knew Basso well, alleged that 'Birillo' was in fact the name of his dog.

The Tour continued, but CSC press conferences took a surreal turn. Questioned repeatedly, Riis and his riders insisted time after time that they did not know the name of Basso's dog. The bags labelled simply 'Jan' proved less of a puzzle – at least as far as T-Mobile's management were concerned.

With characteristic clumsiness, Ullrich, so it seemed, had dug his own hole. T-Mobile claimed he and his coach, Rudy Pevenage, had not told them the truth about their alleged contacts with Fuentes. Presented by the UCI with evidence suggesting that both Pevenage and Ullrich knew Fuentes well and had been in regular contact with the Spaniard, T-Mobile took a hard line and pulled their leader out of the Tour.

'Take a DNA test,' T-Mobile's director of communications Christian Frommert repeatedly told Ullrich. Riis asked Basso to do the same. Both riders refused. Basso remained in Italy crying foul, but 'Ullé's' relationship with T-Mobile was beyond repair. Midway through the 2006 Tour, they sacked him. Six months later, still protesting his innocence, he quit the sport.

Basso spent July 2006 in Italy, smouldering, watching the Tour on his plasma screen, his lawyers talking for him. He would be exonerated, they said. He was innocent of any wrongdoing. Throughout the autumn of 2006, their legal mantras ran along-side those of Tyler Hamilton and, following his positive test, Tour winner, Floyd Landis. They will be exonerated. They are inno-cent. They will ride the Tour again. To date, none of them has.

As winter settled on the Mediterranean, the Spanish investiga-tion was faltering, weighed down by legal procedures, a reluctance on the part of the Spanish judicial system to accelerate the process, and by the clear indication that the Guardia Civil swooped on Saiz and Fuentes too soon. Rumours circulated that no charges would be pressed.

Still, neither Ullrich nor Basso submitted to DNA testing. Their lawyers remained bullish, denouncing the allegations even as the UCI requested more substantial evidence from Madrid so that they could instigate their own investigation. It was not forthcoming.

Despite the pleas of the UCI to await further developments, Ivan Basso was initially cleared of any wrongdoing by CONI, the

Italian Olympic Committee. Perhaps he could go back to CSC and pick up where he left off. But his relationship with Riis, strained by the events of Strasbourg, had become irretrievable. The spell had been broken. He and CSC parted company. So much for the special relationship between the Italian and his Guru.

But Basso had been busy behind the scenes, cultivating another special relationship.

On 8 November, 2006, four months after Johan Bruyneel had lobbied for his expulsion from the Tour de France, Ivan Basso signed a two-year contract with the Discovery Channel team, formerly sponsored by US Postal and part-owned by Lance Armstrong. Both Basso and Bruyneel indicated that, hypothetically, at some time in the future, should he be asked and if it was under the right circumstances, that maybe – just maybe – Ivan would submit to DNA testing.

Riis had supported Basso's suspension because, like most other *directeurs*, he had believed that a gentleman's pact was in place dictating that no ProTour team would hire riders implicated in Operacíon Puerto. Basso's move to Discovery left him in a state of shock.

Suspension by CSC had driven Basso's market value to its lowest level for years, because he was seen as damaged goods. Discovery secured his services at a far cheaper price than if the Italian had raced, and, in all probability, won, the 2006 Tour for Bjarne Riis and CSC. Their decision to sign Basso was widely criticised. Bruyneel, Stapleton and Armstrong, the driving forces behind Tailwind Sports, the management company of the Discovery team, were unperturbed.

Two years late and flying in the face of the post-Puerto ethical pact between the leading teams, and against the wishes of the UCI, Armstrong and Bruyneel finally had their man. Even better, Basso's suspension by CSC in July 2006 – under pressure from, among others, Bruyneel – had actually worked in their favour.

Yet the honeymoon period was short. Basso never raced in anger for Discovery, leaving the team by mutual agreement the following spring, following his confession of 'attempted doping' to CONI. 'Yes, I am Birillo,' he finally admitted, that same sly smile playing on his lips. Basso was banned from racing once more. The Operacíon Puerto investigation, stagnant for more than a year, was finally reopened in February 2008.

Eufemiano Fuentes had worked in cycling for many years, stretching back well before the Festina Affair. His name is well known within the milieu, even if his exact skills remain unclear. The man in the eye of the Operacíon Puerto storm was arrested on 26 May, 2006 and released on bail of 120,0000 euros the following day.

At first Fuentes was indignant over his treatment. Then, unmasked, the 51-year-old became a tabloid celebrity. There he was, scuttling across the tarmac to his plane – the Machiavellian doctor to the stars, unshaven, hiding behind his shades, a bottle of water clutched in one hand, his mobile in the other – looking like the man who broke the bank at Monte Carlo.

He started talking to newspapers and radio stations, defending himself as a 'man of honour'. In an interview with Spanish radio, displaying a little of the boastfulness that tainted Michele Ferrari, he was keen to point out the range of his client base: 'I'm indignant that they're saying that I worked only with cyclists. I've worked with other athletes in athletics, tennis and football.' Maybe, but we have only ever heard about the cyclists.

By December 2006, with the investigation mired in confusion after a series of conflicting rulings in the Spanish courts, there had been little real progress. Nonetheless, Fuentes believed he had become a marked man. He even claimed to have received death threats.

Like Michele Ferrari, Fuentes' comments on doping and ethics only fuelled concerns over the extent of his influence in professional sport. Like Ferrari, Fuentes sought justification by claiming that he had never endangered the health of his clients.

'In twenty-nine years as a professional, none of my clients has had the slightest health problems. I protect the health of the athletes who come to me. Doping is the use or abuse of a substance or medication by somebody who doesn't have the knowledge, experience or skills to use it.

'It's elite sport that is dangerous for the health. It's the overloaded racing calendars and the criminal routes that the organisers design to put on a show that are dangerous,' he said of cycling's European circuit.

Fuentes favoured legalisation of 'therapeutic' doping. 'Doctors must have the freedom and autonomy to be able to decide whether to administer this or that treatment, independent of whether it's doping or not.

'In cycling, they established a maximum haematocrit of fifty per cent, but they never fixed a minimum limit,' he said. 'It's better to ride the Tour de France at fifty-three per cent haematocrit than at thirty-one per cent. Letting a rider take on the Alps with a haematocrit of thirty-one per cent – that's putting his life in danger.'

September 2006, four months after Puerto, and autumn sunshine floods the streets of Salzburg as the World Road Racing Championships take over the city streets. Children dance through the Mirabell flower gardens and onto the Pegasus steps, made famous by *The Sound of Music.* Their parents look down delightedly from the top step, arranging their kids in pecking order, youngest to oldest, ready to be pixelated for their digital memories.

A stone's throw away, across the Mirabellplatz, there is little time for child's play.

Three months after the expiry of his two-year doping ban, David Millar is about to make his comeback for the Great Britain cycling team. Some felt that, in the circumstances, Millar's return was indecently hasty. Not Team GB's pragmatic performance director, David Brailsford, who had supported Millar through his ban and who now welcomed him back with open arms. Two years later, Dwain Chambers became a pariah following his selection for the British team. Millar's return, in contrast, went relatively unnoticed.

David looks as fit as I have ever seen him, lean, focussed and ambitious. Yet among his Great Britain teammates, his rehabilitation creates a sense of unease. Nicole Cooke, firmly established now as Team GB's leading light on the road, struggles to hide her disappointment at his inclusion in the national squad.

In the pit lane, Cooke is warming down after racing in the women's time trial. Experience has taught me that after racing she is usually best left alone for a while before being asked questions. So I bide my time before saying hello and switching on the tape recorder.

'You've been a fierce critic of those riders who've doped in the past, Nicole . . .'

'Well, who wouldn't be?' she snapped back.

Deliberately and carefully choosing her words, she expanded on her theme. 'I really think that if someone makes the conscious decision to dope they also have the choice not to, so once they have had one chance to make a decision and they make the wrong one, then they should pay the consequences.'

So you don't agree with David Millar returning to the British national squad?

'Rules are made – not by myself – and you have to accept the rules. If a time comes post-cycling when I could make some positive changes to the sport then maybe I'd get interested, but I can't change the situation we're in now. So David's here as part of the team . . . and so am I.

'I think David respects me, and I' – she paused – 'I respect . . . the position that David's in. I'm not going to waste time thinking about David's situation and I don't suppose he will spend time thinking about mine.'

Twenty-four hours later, on the finish line of the elite men's time trial, Millar freewheels to a halt and unclips his aerodynamic racing helmet. As he lifts it off his head, a waterfall of sweat cascades down his face and neck.

It hasn't been a vintage performance. He is asked some inane questions. He shrugs and offers deliberately inane answers. The huddle around him disperses and shuffles back across the road to greet the next breathless finisher.

A burly figure strides out of the crowd and embraces him. I crane my neck and recognise Gordon, David's father. They chat briefly and David hugs him goodbye. Then he turns and weaves his way through the crowd and away towards his GB team car, parked discreetly among the deserted backstreets. As he begins to pedal away, I catch his eye.

'Jez – where have you been?' he says.

We chat briefly. He tells me that, in the post-Puerto climate, as one of the few riders willing to discuss doping openly he has 'loads of offers' from other teams. 'Ironic, isn't it,' he says, 'but my PR value is pretty good these days . . .'

So, after he said that, I felt obliged to tell him about the story I'd been working on. Even as David made his comeback from his ban, and with the Puerto scandal raging around the Tour, it emerged that he had been training in Tuscany with Luigi Cecchini, protégé and friend of Conconi and Ferrari, Hamilton and Riis.

In Salzburg, there was confusion over how this alliance began. Millar's new manager, Max Sciandri, now retired from racing, hardly helped things when he gave some awkward justifications to the German press.

'David had some training sessions with Cecchini in May and June in Lucca,' he said. 'It's a delicate issue. David is a pro and I can't tell him what to do. Everybody sets their own limits. I am a friend of Cecchini, but right now there is no relationship between David and Cecchini.'

Sciandri himself, also an adviser to British cycling, is another former protégé of the Tuscan-based Cecchini. Like Conconi and Ferrari, Cecchini is one of the doctors, the mythical figures behind a generation of champions, whose Tuscan treatment rooms transformed careers.

Cecchini, like Ferrari, seemed to inspire intense loyalty. Armstrong never deserted Ferrari, even when – or perhaps because

– most of the media were calling the relationship ill-advised. Tyler Hamilton had a similar attitude towards Cecchini. At the press conference after he won his Olympic gold medal in 2004, the Bostonian called Cecchini a 'second father'.

Millar had first spoken about his contact with Cecchini in July 2006, when talking to British journalists William Fotheringham and Richard Moore. A day before the Salzburg time trial, the connection resurfaced when the German media picked up on the story.

Later, I called David Brailsford, the Team GB manager. At first he was reluctant to elaborate, but then said: 'If Dave had a relationship with Cecchini, we would say thank you and goodbye. I told him he shouldn't have done it and that Team GB don't want to have any association with Cecchini. I have complete confidence in Dave. He knows that in this climate he has to be very careful as to who he associates with.'

Yet a few weeks later, in an interview with French magazine *Velo*, David said that he had worked with Cecchini – with Team GB's knowledge – for three months or so.

'I was clear with Cecchini,' Millar told American journalist James Startt. 'Doping was out of the question. Maybe it was a mistake, but I never hid this collaboration. My federation was aware and I repeat, Cecchini was the first to believe in me.'

So, as David stood there beyond the finish line in Salzburg, I decided to tell him.

'I wrote a story about you and Cecchini,' I said. David nodded. 'I wanted to tell you to your face before anybody else does, or you read about it on the web.'

He nodded again and mumbled something like, 'Fair dos.'

'I just wanted to tell you to your face,' I repeated, hopeful that he would say something that would make me feel less of a Judas.

But he didn't. He just stared past me.

'Yeah, well . . . I better go,' said David and he rode off down the street.

SAVING THE WHALE

January, 2007. Even now, faithless as I am, it's all still so seductive.

In the wind and rain, I catch a flight out to Spain on the day after David Beckham's megadeal with the AEG entertainment group – also owners of the Tour of California bike race – was made public. A few rows in front of me on the plane, Jamie and Louise Redknapp scan the tabloids, as if in disbelief of Goldenballs' Midas touch. We touch down in Majorca on a warm afternoon of long shadows and dappled sunshine.

The next morning, I sit by a cliff-top swimming pool drinking coffee, watching the comings and goings of T-Mobile personnel and guests, as the German sponsor makes ready for its 2007 team launch. The team's management staff of *directeurs* and coaches appears. They are wearing sharp suits and sunglasses, as they line up for yet another photocall. They stand at the edge of the pool, contented smiles and gelled hair. I turn my face upwards for a moment, close my eyes and, after the cold and damp of the English winter, relish the warmth of the sun.

This is the unveiling of the all new T-Mobile cycling team that embraced the changes enforced on them by the fallout from Operacíon Puerto. Jan Ullrich is long gone, but on this glowing January morning, it feels as if the team are breathing a long-awaited sigh of relief and relishing his absence. They have a new team boss, Bob Stapleton. The youthful 47-year-old multi-millionaire, who rides his bike almost every day, bounds on stage at the team presentation and tells anybody who will listen that T-Mobile 'believes in clean and fair sport'. The 'new' T-Mobile, says the press release, 'wants to be a team that fans like, believe in, and ultimately trust.'

In the past, Majorca's Club Robinson, tucked away in the far south-east of the island on the Cala Serena bay, became Club Ullrich for ten days or so. The grounds would be overrun by German tabloid journalists and camera crews, desperate for images that captured Ullrich in the throes of his annual fight against the flab. After a misspent winter, Ullrich was sometimes so unfit that he was unable to train with his teammates. He'd be reduced to huffing and puffing in the slipstream of a team car for hours on end. These sessions often degenerated into farce, as paparazzi motorbikes choked the roads and sparred for shots of a heavy-jowled 'Kaiser' playing catch-up with his fitness. He would amaze us all, months later, when, skin taut on his bones, he lined up for his annual showdown with Lance Armstrong at the Tour.

Stapleton was not the only one in Majorca extolling the virtues of change. His fine words were supported by Christian Prudhomme, the new director of the Tour de France.

Prudhomme's presence was a ringing endorsement of T-Mobile's brave new world. 'We've never seen what happened in Strasbourg in any other sports,' Prudhomme said. 'Don't forget that Operación Puerto has links to football as well – and what did they write about that? Just a line or two!'

Stapleton, less than six months into his new role, looked on as Prudhomme talked to the press. The wiry Californian, made rich by his skills in the telecommunication business, had set about ridding the team of the old cliques. A pragmatist with a ready smile and a firm handshake, he was a good talker at ease with the media.

Stapleton had cleared out the dead wood, or so we thought. He said the right things about the need to combat doping. But there was general bemusement when, following Discovery Channel's capture of Ivan Basso, T-Mobile broke ranks with the other ProTour teams and their gentleman's agreement not to sign any of those alleged to be involved with Puerto, by making a bid for Spaniard Alejandro Valverde.

Perhaps fortunately for Stapleton's brave new world, the deal failed to come off. 'I'm not a diplomat,' he smiled as we sat talking by Club Robinson's pool on another perfect Majorcan morning. 'My friends laugh at me when I'm caught in the middle.'

THE AMERICAN'S FRIENDS

Bob Stapleton was T-Mobile's clean-up man, but he was also a member of a discreet and informal stateside organisation of silver-haired but cycling-mad CEOs called the Champions Club. The Champions Club get-togethers are a far cry from the Sunday club runs of Catford CC or the Merseyside Wheelers. Membership requires a $100,000 admission fee, which may explain why the Champions Club has a limited number of members. It is perhaps the wealthiest cycling club in the world with several members appearing in *Forbes* rich lists. No wonder American commentators had taken to calling cycling 'the new golf'.

The members of the Champions Club are among road cycling's new elite, the super-rich. They have little time for century-old European tradition. Robson Walton, one of the family that own K Mart, Bennett Dorrance, the heir to the Campbell's soup kingdom, George Battle, formerly executive chairman of Internet search engine Ask Jeeves, and Hollywood actor Robin Williams, a close friend of Armstrong, have all ridden with the Champions Club.

One of the club's early members, Ed McCall, first discovered cycling at the 1999 Tour de France. As Lance rode towards his first success, McCall ended up working as an impromptu body-guard for the Texan.

'Knocking these French photographers on their ass,' he told *Outside* magazine, 'was a blast.' The luckier members of the Champions Club get to hang out with Lance and, every now and then, even to ride with him.

Williams, star of *The World According to Garp*, was one of the principal cheerleaders in The World According to Lance. The Hairiest Man in Hollywood was always good copy, and was the most high profile of America's new cycling superfans. He was a regular VIP guest at the finish of the Tour in Paris, where he held court as Lance sealed another success. Gales of indulgent laughter rippled outwards from the huddle around him as the demob-happy peloton tore up and down the Champs-Elysées.

We'd interviewed him for *procycling* when he had been on set in Alaska with Al Pacino making the thriller *Insomnia*. In a bid to make Williams feel more at home, we detailed the effervescent Andy Hood, at that time in London, to the interview. We gathered around, switched on the speakerphone and sat back as Hood jauntily cried: 'Hey Robin! It's Andy Hood here in London.' Between takes, Williams' deep, disembodied voice floated down the phone line. It was like interviewing sixteen different people. Within seconds, Hood was doubled up in mirth, gripped by hysteria, clutching his sides, dropping the phone, stamping the floor. A torrent of accents and mimicry cascaded down the line. Effortlessly, Williams switched from one persona to the next. Listening in wasn't, in truth, that funny. It was uneasy listening. What was funnier was watching Hood dissolve.

Williams did gay Floridian pet-shop owner: 'Oh ex*cuuuu*se me, Mr Armstrong sir, but how often do you shave your legs?' Hood cackled and snorted.

Williams did enraged Texan redneck: 'Boy, dem Lycra shorts look too dang tight to me . . .' Hood's shoulders shook uncontrollably.

Williams did crazed Italian sports doctor: 'Signor Ferrari meet Signor Cecchini, Signor Punto meet Signor Tipo . . .' Tears rolled down Hood's cheeks and he slammed his palm into the desk in submission.

The monologue echoed through the office for thirty minutes until Hood finally managed to splutter 'Thank you, Robin' and put the phone down. It had been a virtuoso performance. We used the cover line 'Lance says I'm bike-sexual'.

Williams may have been the best-known member of the Champions Club, but perhaps the most influential is Thomas Weisel, an investment banker from San Francisco, whose most successful speculation was on a former cancer sufferer and apparently washed-up cyclist called Lance.

Weisel looms large over the recent revolution in American cycling. He founded and funded the team that became US Postal, and he hired its two most high-profile riders, Armstrong and Tyler Hamilton. When Armstrong couldn't get a sponsor after his recovery from cancer, Weisel took the Texan on, but only after striking a hard bargain and telling the Texan to sharpen up his act and start behaving like a real captain of industry.

'He hadn't been enough of a leader,' Weisel has said. 'He was not very respectful of other riders and the support system around him.' For once, Lance was contrite. It was, he said later, 'probably the most brutal conversation I've ever had'.

Weisel is the alpha male of the Champions Club. He appears to be just as driven as Armstrong, perhaps because Weisel's relationship with his father mirrored Lance's own troubled childhood. Weisel wrote in *Capital Instincts*, his autobiography published in 2003, that his father used a stick for 'beating the shit' out of him. Both men like having the odds stacked against them.

Between them, Weisel and Armstrong had changed Middle America's perception of road cycling. They made it appear aspirational, healthy and intelligent. Middle-aged cycling fans don't have to be tubby, balding Europeans in Lycra plodding their way slowly through the Alps or Dolomites, but can instead be silver-haired CEOs with white teeth, tight abs and an SUV support vehicle, touring Colorado or Tuscany.

Weisel is passionate about cycling. He brought a corporate intelligence to a sport that used to be sponsored by shopkeepers and car salesmen. He is a fixer, a dynamic money man with an obsessive's eye. If he sees something is wrong, he has to wade in, straighten it out, do it his way. That was the case with the American national federation, USA Cycling.

Since he dug it out of the red in 2000, USA Cycling has been made in Weisel's image. He shored up their cash crisis with an injection of his own. He also brought in some of his own people who saw things the Weisel Way. This later led to accusations of Weisel as self-serving.

One such character was Steve Johnson, who was brought in as CEO of USA Cycling. Bob Stapleton said that Johnson and Weisel went back a long way. Unsurprising perhaps, then, that Johnson sprung to the defence of fellow Weisel protégé, Champions Club icon and Discovery Channel team owner Lance Armstrong, when in 2005 *L'Equipe* alleged that Armstrong had EPO in his blood during the 1999 Tour. Despite USA Cycling's important role as a disciplinary body over doping violations, Johnson gave the French allegations extremely short shrift.

'This is an issue for the French people,' Johnson told Reuters. 'They seemed very concerned about it, and frankly I don't care what they think. And I don't think Lance does either. This is just a publication in a French tabloid newspaper. That's our perspective.'

Other Weisel acolytes assumed key roles within USA Cycling. Jim Ochowicz, another long-time friend, associate and coach of Armstrong (and Tyler Hamilton and Floyd Landis) – and a broker for Thomas Weisel Partners – became president of USA Cycling.

Ousted by the Weisel regime was Johnson's predecessor as USA Cycling CEO, Gerard Bisceglia – fired by Ochowicz and USA Cycling's board in 2006. I first met Bisceglia at the World Track Championships in Los Angeles in 2005. A burly, immediately likable man, Bisceglia gave me a ride from the Home Depot velodrome – a stone's throw from David Beckham's new home at the LA Galaxy stadium – to the Long Beach Sheraton, where we were both staying.

On the drive across LA, we talked about a young American

rider who had been made offers by several ProTour teams. Bisceglia had doping on his mind. He was anxious that the rider had made the right choice. As he pulled up outside the hotel, the conversation moved on to Tyler Hamilton's choices, for better or worse.

'Seemed such a good kid,' Bisceglia said, shaking his head in dismay.

'You feel pretty strongly about doping then?' I ventured.

'You bet,' he said. 'When I talk to younger riders, I tell them, "If you dope, I will fucking kill you . . ."'

After he retired from racing, Frankie Andreu became part of the USA Cycling establishment. Andreu had enjoyed a respectable, if low-key, career, with Motorola, Cofidis and US Postal. Much of his racing had been spent working for his team leader and close friend, Lance Armstrong. Outwardly, Andreu had long appeared to be a bastion of the Texan's clan, but Frankie had a guilty conscience that he could not ignore. Eventually, it over-powered him.

In 2006, supported by his wife Betsy, he confessed to doping himself with EPO while racing as Armstrong's teammate. Maybe, if he hadn't been subpoenaed and definitively opposed Lance as a result of the SCA investigation, maybe if he'd been kept close to the Texan and his entourage rather than slowly exiled, things would have been different. Maybe then Frankie would have kept his mouth shut, just as he had done after retiring from racing in December 2000 and taking up a job in TV, his years on the road, bitching about the hotels, the food, the travelling, finally behind him.

But then, as he watched his old friend Lance become an icon and his former teammates get richer, the years spent as cannon fodder in the peloton stuck in his throat. So when Juliet Macur of the *New York Times* stood in his kitchen and asked, out of the blue, 'Frankie – did you dope?' he couldn't hold back any more. Frankie gave her a straight answer. 'Yes,' he said.

When the *New York Times* ran their story there was another anonymous confession alongside Frankie's; that of one of his US Postal teammates from 1999.

It had happened, they both said, in 1999, training for the Tour – in Andreu's case, he said, EPO injections, three times. Frankie may have been a great *domestique*, but he was never good enough to win any big European races. So he had specialised in helping others, particularly his friend Lance, to win – and to win big. In the press room, 'Crankie Frankie' had a reputation as a bullshit-free zone, unpretentious, pragmatic, straight-talking – and on occasion, downright rude.

But this time, the more he talked, the more damaging his words became. Like so many others, Andreu had respected the *omerta*. Like so many others, he'd just been 'doing his job', being a good pro, by embracing the simple and readily available deceit of doping. That was why it came as such a shock when he decided to tell the truth. His confession, six years after his retirement, was totally unexpected.

Frankie said he felt little fear of either the doping controls or the haematocrit check as he topped up his blood.

'The controls just said stay below fifty per cent. That was what much of the peloton had been doing for years. But I wasn't trying to approach those levels – I was just trying to feel *normal* in the peloton again.'

He had learned about the powers of EPO and its use through 'gossip, the papers, magazines. It was a very hot topic during the 1990s,' he said. There was, he says, no peer pressure. 'My job would be on the line if I didn't perform but that was the case for everyone. I had internal pressure that I put on myself. I knew there were riders taking EPO before I did, but it's an individual choice in the end.'

He denied that there was a structured culture of doping within the US Postal team. 'On any team, anybody who did anything did it individually, so there was no way of knowing if anybody else was doing anything. I'm speaking about personal choices that I made. I was not put under pressure or told to do it.' Frankie said that EPO gave him an amazing improvement in performance. He estimated that using it made him perform 'twenty per cent better' as a professional athlete. 'I was able to be a bike racer again instead of being a pack filler.'

So why, after all these years, had he decided to confess? What was the point? 'Because of what has been going on in the sport,' he replied. 'I realised that I had done something wrong in the past too, and that I couldn't speak freely or feel good about it until I admitted that I got caught up in it. I was asked point blank if I did it and I thought, "It's time to make a decision here. Now's the time to stop covering up things, to stop lying and to tell the truth." So I answered the question truthfully.

'There's been no closure to a lot of these cases. People keep denying and lying. So I'm trying to change that.'

Johan Bruyneel, his old team manager at US Postal, was not impressed. The Belgian described Andreu's admission as 'pitiful'. Frankie was not surprised by Bruyneel's reaction.

'I was disappointed that he made that remark instead of looking at the positive side of trying to clean up the sport and of trying to make the sport better. Obviously, he only thinks about himself and his team. Johan Bruyneel is in charge of himself, so he can live with his words.'

Andreu's confession split the US Cycling community. While some, like Bisceglia, were sympathetic, others condemned him. 'I expected some negative reaction,' Frankie says, 'because what I did was wrong, but the positive responses were overwhelming. People are sick of the deceit so I think it was a refreshing change for the truth to come out.

'I had some positive response from riders. Anybody who gives me a negative response is missing the point. I truly believe that every single rider racing now would like to be able to race clean.'

The US Postal team's management company, Tailwind Sports,

co-owned by Thom Weisel and Armstrong – both, like Andreu, in senior positions within the USA Cycling hierarchy – reacted strongly and lobbied for sanctions against their former employee.

'Team management will be investigating this issue and considering all legal options and trust that the relevant authorities (USA Cycling, USADA and the UCI) will be doing the same,' said a press release.

Meanwhile, Bisceglia, who worked with Andreu during their time together at USA Cycling, watched developments from his home in Colorado.

'Frankie's a retired rider – what are you gonna do to him? I like Frankie. I never doubted any of the things he told me. I was disappointed and shocked when I heard about his admission of EPO use. Not in him, but in the sport, because I thought of him as one of the good guys.'

Bisceglia knew that Andreu had nothing to gain by coming clean. 'He'll pay a heavy price for his admission; this code of silence, the *omerta*,' he said scornfully, 'it's like the Mafia . . . what does that tell you about the sport?'

Yet it was the banality of Andreu's confession that was its most shocking characteristic. EPO had not made him into a champion, but merely helped him survive. Even with a twenty per cent lift to his performance, his best results from his EPO season are hardly memorable. In 1999, he finished in twenty-first place at both Paris–Roubaix and the Tour of Luxembourg, his highest finishes of the season. He placed sixty-fifth in that year's Tour de France and would have received a share of Armstrong's winnings for overall victory.

Nonetheless, reaching for the syringe had got to him. 'It was on my conscience, but I was only trying to keep up by doing what everybody else was doing. Once I retired from racing, I didn't really think about it until I had to start speaking about it, and it seemed to be a continuing problem in the peloton.

'People say, "Why bring up the past?" But I'm bringing up

the past to be able to clean up the present. It got to the point where the problem got out of control. Now we're struggling to get things back to a clean sport. Riders want to race clean. They don't like the fact they may have to dope to race or that the sport is known to be so dirty.'

He believes that there is plenty of doping still going on. 'As things stand now a rider can micro-dose, which means that they can take just a little bit of something, to stay out of that huge window that is the positive area,' he said.

In the United States, Andreu's confession was read by some – including Armstrong himself – as a direct implication of his former team leader and estranged friend.

His relationship with Armstrong has only gone backwards since Andreu took the decision to testify in the SCA arbitration case. Even though he and Lance were once 'very good friends' while racing together, they have become estranged over the past few years.

'We lived together for a while in Italy, although once I retired we drifted a little bit apart, but we were still friends. Then the Walsh book came out, and the SCA case came out and things fell apart very quickly. I didn't talk to Lance for about two and a half years,' Frankie recalls.

Lance had kept his phone number, though. 'When I got subpoenaed for the SCA case, the day before I was deposed, he phoned me up, out of the blue. I was very surprised by that.'

Andreu and his wife, Betsy, told the SCA arbitration hearings that in 1996, when being treated for cancer in hospital, Armstrong had, in their presence, told doctors that he had used doping products. Armstrong, and other witnesses who were present at the time, gave evidence and denied that he ever said this.

Frankie and Lance, once seemingly inseparable, were now on opposite sides of cycling's great divide. 'It didn't bother me – I was living my life, he was living his life, and I was fine with our paths not crossing again, but then the SCA case made things a lot more difficult. Lance really attacked my wife's character and my character. I didn't appreciate that, so there's no love lost for him now.'

In the aftermath of his confession, Andreu says it was quietly suggested to him that he might like to resign from his role at USA Cycling. 'I declined,' he said. He knows that he might yet suffer the same fate as those who went before him, shouting their mouths off about doping. He may join others, such as Christophe Bassons and Filippo Simeoni, in no-man's-land.

For the moment, his resolve is holding firm. Perhaps it helps that, unlike Simeoni, he is no longer fighting to hold down a professional contract with an elite European team. He remains involved in cycling, though, as a coach and TV pundit.

'I always thought highly of Simeoni. The guy's never really done anything wrong. Armstrong was the one who was very aggressive towards him. I didn't doubt anything that Simeoni said.

'I remember Christophe Bassons speaking out. Again, the guy who went after him was Lance. I don't think there were many other riders who went after him and attacked him – it was just Lance,' Frankie said. 'Lance went after Simeoni, Lance went after Bassons.'

And, I say to him, it turns out Bassons and Simeoni were right: doping was still an issue in 1999, because Frankie and his anonymous teammate had used EPO and look, it was still an issue in 2004, because Frankie's ex-teammate, Tyler Hamilton, another of the US Postal class of '99, got busted for blood transfusions. And it was still an issue in early 2008, when his old boss, Johan Bruyneel, found his Astana team blackballed from every significant professional event.

Frankie reflects on that thought for a moment. 'In a way, maybe I'm lucky, because I didn't mess around with all that stuff for a long period. But,' he says, 'a lot of other riders did.'

★   ★   ★

Bob Stapleton may have been a member of the Champion's Club, but he believed he was not compromised by past relationships.

'I don't have any ties that stop me from saying what I think,' he maintained, as we sat talking in the Spanish sunshine. I never doubted that Stapleton meant what he said. It's just that I was not convinced that he fully understood the nature of what he was dealing with.

All that stuff about 'cleaning up the sport' – they said all the same things after the Festina Affair, and look at what had happened since then. So why should we believe it now? Why should T-Mobile be different to the others and to what has gone before?

Stapleton had come on board to restore T-Mobile's credibility, but the key to the continuation of the sponsorship lay in results. T-Mobile is a big global brand – it is not T-Mobile Milan, T-Mobile United, or T-Mobile Madrid, built on a sense of place or a loyal fan base; this multimillion-euro sponsorship was about selling, and to sell, the team needs results.

Stapleton nodded and listened. But he sounded as if he was shooting for the stars when he said that 'what's different is that T-Mobile is now a like-minded group of managers, athletes and sponsors, focussed on the mission. We consciously went through a clean-out – we changed most of our people – and now we have over twenty-five new people in terms of management and athletes. We have a medical advisory board that makes sure that all of our methods are the best, both in terms of anti-doping and in terms of athlete development.'

A reliance on doping, he argued, is based on ignorance. 'The philosophy behind doping starts with thinking that everybody is doing it, that to be on a level playing field it's necessary, and that you're disadvantaged if you don't do it. But in many cases the riders have very little information. They hear things, they're told things by people that seem influential and once they start, it's a very slippery slope. It's very hard to change. The psychology of doping is treacherous.'

Team insiders said that T-Mobile came within a hair's breadth of pulling out of cycling when the sky fell in Strasbourg and Ullrich's reputation collapsed. The spin was that the sponsor had stayed to clean things up and to set a good example. Even so, there were still riders in T-Mobile's squad whose good intentions had been questioned in the past. Giuseppe Guerini, tormentor of Filippo Simeoni, was still there, as was multiple world champion Michael Rogers, whose working relationship – although terminated – with Michele Ferrari became public knowledge during the 2006 Tour.

Stapleton continued, explaining that the riders would adhere to a new, more personalised training regime and follow a daily 'Pillar Strength' routine with a team of American fitness specialists who had also worked with Jurgen Klinsmann's highly successful German national football team. But I sat there thinking, that's great – and where will they get that extra twenty per cent that Frankie Andreu believed EPO gave him? From a Pillar Strength routine?

'We definitely have athletes who have come because they are fed up and they want to be in an environment where they feel they can develop naturally and there is no pressure. If we can bring some fresh clean faces that have a commitment to anti-doping we will regain public interest.'

It was a stirring speech.

When he ended it, despite my misgivings, I was, for a brief moment, up there with Bob Stapleton, flying the flag, waving to the cheering crowds, imagining that bright new tomorrow, free of the syringes and the *omerta* and the bitterness, embracing that new dawn that cycling so desperately needed.

I walked away with a spring in my step and a warm and sunny feeling towards my fellow man. But then I heard Kimmage's voice telling me, 'No second chances . . .' and then Lance's voice, growling about 'protecting the interests of the peloton', and I checked myself and realised that it was really not as simple as Bob Stapleton imagined it was.

And then I remembered that the last time I'd felt the same 'we are the world' glow was when the northern bottlenose whale was winched out of the Thames, with people cheering from the riverbank in Battersea Park and the collective love of the British capital willing it to survive. But the whale died.

Stapleton had talked of creating a 'clean and fair' team, one that could win from March until October. The big question as the minivans ferried the press back to Palma airport, was could T-Mobile's riders achieve results if they were all, as he insisted, clean?

Sitting beside me in the departure lounge, a German journalist poured scorn on T-Mobile's transformation under Stapleton. 'How can they win any races without doping, without any leaders, when other teams are doping?' he said. 'This is PR bullshit. It won't work.'

After Operacíon Puerto cut a swathe through the starters at the 2006 Tour de France, there was a notion, based on little more than a feel-good factor, that the race was somehow purged of doping.

On the night before his victory parade on the Champs-Elysées, Floyd Landis didn't want to talk about doping. 'Got any other questions?' he snapped, at the winner's press conference, when Operacíon Puerto became the main theme. The sentiment that, with the Fuentes network in disarray, it had been a cleaner Tour, didn't last long. Two nights after I got home from Paris, the biggest story of all broke.

Late in the evening, I stood in my back garden, mobile pressed to my ear. Music was blaring from an open window on the other side of the wall. My phone beeped ominously as the battery ran down.

'You're sure? At Morzine? It's definitely Floyd?'

The voice at the other end of the phone, speaking softly from a deserted office block in central Paris, assured me again that it was indeed Floyd Landis who had tested positive for testosterone, just two days after celebrating victory in the 2006 Tour de France.

'*Ouai . . . c'est sur.* Jeremy – yes.'

'*D'accord, merci.* Thank you – *à bientôt.*'

My phone beeped once more and then went dead.

I ran inside, grabbed my wife's phone and called the UCI president, Pat McQuaid.

I apologised for calling so late and then in the same breath said: 'The positive – it's Landis, isn't it?'

He wouldn't confirm or deny the rumours.

But he did say this: 'I'm extremely angry. The credibility of the sport is at stake. It's the worst-case scenario.'

And after Pat McQuaid had said that, I knew that it just had to be Floyd.

As he has got older, Greg LeMond has become increasingly outspoken. At first he was discreet about his opinions; now he shouts them from the rooftops.

'I told Floyd Landis the other day,' he was saying, 'I want to believe that I would have been somebody who was strong enough to say no, but I can't be sure of that because I didn't come into cycling in 1993, 1994, 1995, when blood doping was rampant. I didn't have to make that choice.'

LeMond has been through the mill over the past few years. He has been tested by dark secrets from his childhood, by his son's addiction problems, by his own reliance on alcohol – now a thing of the past, he says – and by the strain all of this has put on his marriage to Kathy.

A few months after the news over Floyd's positive test broke, Greg spoke to him on the phone. LeMond recalled the conversation. 'He'd got two positive tests for synthetic testosterone out of one sample, and I was just saying, "*Please* – don't do a Tyler Hamilton."'

Landis was taken aback by LeMond's advice. Immediately afterwards, his strict upbringing in the obscure and separatist

Mennonite religion showed when he told an Internet forum that he would rather 'talk to Satan before Greg LeMond'.

When I interviewed him over email, Landis explained further: 'Greg basically told the press that I called him and admitted that I had doped. No such thing ever happened. I was legitimately upset when I made that comment on the forum,' he told me.

LeMond scorned Landis' anger. 'I've gone through my own personal change in the last three or four years and have looked at myself in terms of who I am. I didn't want to upset anybody. I always wanted people to like me, but that was at a personal cost to me. I let people take advantage of me. I've decided to stand up for my own principles, regardless of whether it's unpopular or not.'

Landis also wrote on his website, 'If I reveal what Greg told me, it would destroy his character.'

LeMond insisted that he was only trying to save Landis from the pain of living a lie. 'I told Floyd that I'd lived with a secret for most of my life and it almost destroyed my marriage.' He paused. 'The secret was that I was sexually abused before I got into cycling.

'I felt bad for Floyd – he'd been writing the most disgusting mean things about me, comparing me to Satan. I was trying to tell him, that if he did indeed take testosterone, that to go on having to defend yourself and live in fear of somebody finding out that you really did cheat, that the cost emotionally is so much greater than the short-term shame and embarrassment of coming clean.

'I'm not a saint,' Greg continued. 'I've got stuff in my life, in my past that on a personal level I am not proud of, but I am human and we all have flaws. The fact that I can tell you about being abused – I mean, four years ago I couldn't even tell my wife without a bottle of Scotch in me. But I was really forced to face it because I was going to lose my family.'

Poor Floyd. What a catastrophe winning the Tour was for him. For those who cheered him on, from disastrous failure to heroic comeback, who supported him to 'victory', the sense of waste was equally overpowering – wasted time, wasted hopes, wasted effort.

I had never warmed to Landis. I first spoke to him one spring evening long ago when he was racing for the ill-fated Mercury team, ironically on LeMond-branded bikes. He was sitting on the edge of the curb outside the team hotel. He'd been friendly enough. But, once into the US Postal bubble, in the orbit of Armstrong and Bruyneel, his head seemed to be turned.

On *procycling*, we'd developed a habit of picking out new talent, rather than sticking to the same old faces. Landis hadn't won any big races, but he had attitude and stood out from the crowd. And he was a little intriguing too, his quaint turn of phrase, a hangover from his strictly religious upbringing, now punctuated by good ol' boy characteristics, such as his penchant for ZZ Top.

But with attitude and ego came petulance. Floyd had a tendency to sulk, when things didn't work out. On the 2004 Paris-Nice, he finished third on the stage to Gap. Not such a blow you might think, but he stomped into the team bus in a huff and wouldn't come to the door to talk to a handful of journalists waiting in the rain.

A couple of days later, as the teams lined up on the promenade des Anglais on the final morning of the race in Nice, I decided to try again. I bounded up to him, exchanged greetings, and then said, as we had said to others before him: 'We want to put you on the cover of *procycling* magazine!'

Normally, the rider's face lit up. Not Floyd's. He was sullen and unimpressed. 'Talk to my agent,' he said bluntly and rode off down the boulevard.

He could be as graceless in victory as he was in defeat. In his Tour winner's press conference, two years later, the evening before his victory parade in Paris, as the repercussions of Operacíon Puerto swirled around the race, he opted to play dumb.

Did he think that Puerto, which even Lance Armstrong, Landis' mentor and former team captain, had described as 'probably the biggest scandal since the Festina Affair', and the absence of Ullrich and Basso devalued his Tour win?

'I don't know anything about that,' he said.

Somebody asked him again: 'Look, as you keep asking, I'll say that it was an unfortunate situation and none of us got any satisfaction out of the fact that they weren't here – got any questions about anything else?'

Floyd was the latest ex-US Postal rider to emerge from the shadow of Lance with a depressing story: a career-threatening illness or injury, a heroic comeback, followed swiftly by an indignant fan-based crusade to fight the injustice of the doping allegations made against him.

Floyd's immediate predecessor was Tyler Hamilton, who rode a whole Tour with a broken collarbone yet still might have won the race. But Floyd's against-all-odds story was perhaps the more extreme, as he won the world's hardest bike race on one leg, due to a degenerative hip injury.

Both Hamilton and Landis adhered to the same blueprint. Hamilton fought a long battle to clear his name of blood doping, at one point citing a disappearing twin in his mother's womb. 'Maybe he should hire an exorcist,' Dick Pound said. Landis, humiliated within hours of celebrating his 2006 Tour win, blamed a mid-Tour bender and came up with the 'Whiskey Defence'.

In fact, the alarm bells about Landis were ringing long before he won the 2006 Tour. Halfway through the race, he held a press conference and decided to tell the world about his crumbling hip joint, damaged in a training crash while with US Postal a couple of years earlier. He had a therapeutic exemption to take cortisone from the UCI; effectively a licence to take drugs to counter the pain of his hip injury.

In the end, though, it wasn't the cortisone that caught up with him, but the testosterone. So when in July 2006, 'Floyd the Void' tested positive and came tumbling down from his perch, blaming the whiskey, blaming the French lab, there was little sympathy for him. At least, not from me.

Call it *Schadenfreude*, or maybe just call it compassion fatigue. There's no doubt that his career was ruined by the ensuing scandal. But then, a part of me thinks that Floyd Landis, however intelligent, got what he and his fucked-up, hypocritical, self-serving ethos really deserved.

After he tested positive, Floyd Landis fought back. And in doing so he made things much worse for everybody.

His positive test, hot on the heels of Puerto, may have been the 'worst-case scenario' for the UCI and the Tour, but the real nadir came in the late spring of 2007, when paedophilia, doping and witness intimidation became the currency of the Landis doping hearing in Malibu, California.

Landis had spent months protesting his innocence. He had launched the Floyd Fairness Fund, attracting huge donations from supportive fans, claiming that the case wasn't really about him, but about the integrity of anti-doping; he had attacked WADA and their protocols and accused the French anti-doping lab in Châtenay-Malabry of incompetence and bias. Yet the two positive tests for synthetic testosterone still hung over his head.

So the Landis camp tried a new tactic. The night before Greg LeMond was due to appear as a witness against Landis, Will Geoghegan, Landis' business manager and an active fundraiser for the Floyd Fairness Fund, called LeMond and impersonated the uncle who had sexually abused him as a child.

The call left LeMond in a state of shock, but through the police he traced it back to Geoghegan's cellphone. The next morning, as he gave evidence, LeMond held up his BlackBerry with Geoghegan's number clearly displayed. The Landis team held their heads in their hands. Geoghegan promptly apologised but Landis sacked his business manager on the spot. A day later, it was announced that Geoghegan had gone into rehab, after claiming that, unprompted by Landis, he had only called LeMond in a drunken rage. Once again, the booze was to blame.

It's to his credit that Greg LeMond still describes Floyd Landis as 'a good guy', well educated and decent. He considers Tyler Hamilton in the same light. 'I don't believe Tyler is some kind of thief who would cheat or steal normally. But it's the culture of the sport that convinces an ethical normal person that this is what you have to do.'

It's well over twenty years since LeMond became the first American to win the Tour de France. It's a decade since 1998, when doping first threatened to destroy the race, a scandal that fuelled the formation of WADA. From Festina to Floyd, LeMond agrees that little about cycling's culture has really changed.

'Lance always says that it's the people who speak out who are destroying the sport. No − it's the cheats who are destroying the sport. I'm not destroying it by speaking out, nor is Christophe Bassons, nor Filippo Simeoni or anybody else who speaks out. Because,' says Greg LeMond, 'if you can't recognise there's a problem, then you never cure the problem.'

GRILLING THE CHICKEN

Michael Rasmussen cocked his bald, sculpted head and anxiously eyed the audience of journalists dissecting his every word.

There were plenty of questions. There were questions about what he had told his team, Rabobank, about his whereabouts in the build-up to the 2007 Tour de France, questions about what he had told the UCI, questions about why he had missed four out-of-competition doping tests, questions about why he, as a Dane, seemed so determined to avoid taking out a racing licence in his home country, where anti-doping had become a burning issue.

It all came down to trust.

'Yes – you can trust me,' Rasmussen told the media in response to a question from Lars Werge, the equally bald, equally sculpted, and deeply inquisitive journalist from *Ekstra Bladet* in Denmark.

The towering, softly-spoken Werge was Rasmussen's principal inquisitor. A former international high jumper turned journalist, Lars has the languid limbs of a giraffe and the cranium of the Mekon. Naturally, his physique made him unmissable, as he strolled between team cars and buses in start villages and finish areas, scrutinising the world from behind his Ray-Bans. Lars stood out. He was lofty enough to shade under on a hot afternoon.

During the 2001 Tour, his giraffe-like physique had even alarmed the implacable Armstrong. One morning we gathered around the doors of the US Postal bus. Lance dutifully appeared and we crowded around him. Lars asked him questions about the latest doping allegations. Not for the first time, he patted them away as old, dead, meaningless, but then concluded by rather smugly telling Lars, 'You'd understand that – if you had ever been an elite athlete.'

Lars paused and glowered at the Texan. He craned his elastic neck and leaned closer to Armstrong. 'Actually, Lance,' he hissed, 'I was.' Armstrong was soon back in the bus.

Now, with the Alpine stages of the 2007 Tour de France looming on the horizon and Rasmussen moving into contention for victory, Werge had to make a choice. Could Rasmussen be trusted? The 'Chicken', as the pale and pasty Rasmussen was nicknamed, had been anonymous since the London prologue. Now, he was ready to challenge. But his twitchy and uneasy appearances before the media only enhanced the impression of an athlete with something to hide.

Ten days earlier, Rasmussen's name had gone unnoticed. As the teams gathered in London for the start of the 2007 Tour, the focus had been on Vinokourov, Riis, Kasechkin, and, of course, Ferrari, as Ken Livingstone's attempts to force Londoners to embrace his two-wheeled Utopia were washed away by grey skies, foul-mouthed builders and doping, doping – always doping.

Fighting to hold on to his dream of success in the Tour's London prologue, on a route that mapped out his life story, Bradley Wiggins found himself assailed by feature writers telling him that cycling was a dirty, dead-end sport. Unsurprisingly, after weeks of defending his sport, he was in a grump. Like others, he seemed exhausted and wrung out by the constant questions on drugs. To make things worse, 'Wiggo' had been abused by white van man while out training with his Cofidis teammates.

Even prior to that, he wasn't speaking to many people, least of all me. A little problem had surfaced between us in the build-up to the Tour. He felt that something I'd written had betrayed his trust. That misunderstanding culminated in him sending me an angry text message.

I liked Bradley – we had even ridden the prologue route together.

But then I wrote a speculative news story, legitimately quoting his team manager Eric Boyer as saying that he might be dropped from the Cofidis team for the Tour unless his results picked up.

Now if you talk to those who know the Olympic gold medal-list well, they will shrug and say, 'So what – he didn't call you back. It's happened before.' But Bradley seemed such a decent bloke, bitterly outspoken about doping, and one of the few riders that I could still feel some kinship with. I hated the notion that he thought I was trying to undermine him.

Wiggins was one of the riders championed as having un-impeachable integrity and credibility – even Kimmage agreed on that. But he blew hot and cold and getting to know him well was a tall order, given his mercurial nature. Only a couple of journalists had really achieved this. But then, perhaps because of some remnants of my own youthful confusion, I had always felt drawn to the anti-Wig – David Millar.

Bradley thawed a little when we met again. 'I thought you were stirring it,' he said, with a wry smile. But as London's poster boy for the Tour's visit, there was no doubt that he was feeling the pressure of expectation of the opening weekend. Millar, in contrast, had been left to his own devices, a reformed doper coming to terms with the realities of racing in front of home crowds. But, holed up in his hotel, under the lattice of flyovers and interchanges criss-crossing London's Docklands, the matured Millar, the reborn, evangelical Millar, was having trouble making his voice heard.

There had been gossip about tensions in his relationship with his sponsor Saunier Duval and about his relationship with the team manager, Mauro Gianetti. The rumour, that it had been over the bad habits of some of his teammates and about David's readiness to condemn doping, had taken hold in the press room. There had been a row and Millar, the story went, had even written to the UCI to see if he could escape the team. Had it really got that bad?

We sat beneath the flyovers, chatting in the coffee bar of the

Docklands Crowne Plaza. 'Cycling is a complete mess at the moment and it's been building up for years,' Millar said. 'It's going to get worse before it gets better.'

Across the car park, Wiggins and his Cofidis teammates climbed aboard their bike-laden team coach and headed out towards the M25 to train in the quieter lanes of Essex. We watched them leave. Everything had been sorted out with Mauro, Millar said. The disagreement had been resolved. Yet that lunchtime, when his teammates took to the streets, Millar was an exception, opting to train on his stationary bike in the hotel car park.

As I was leaving, Gianetti strolled over and presented him with a new aerodynamic time-trial helmet, emblazoned not only with the Union Jack, but also with an image of Millar in the playboy days of his youth, clutching two glasses of frothing beer. It was flash, but it wasn't the older, wiser David that I now knew. On the day of the prologue, Millar didn't wear it.

Back in the press room, I called Pat McQuaid, who confirmed that Millar had written to him about his worries over doping. 'They were emails discussing anti-doping in general,' McQuaid told me. I told McQuaid of my sense of Millar's isolation within his team. He listened.

'Any rider who is being victimised because of his stance on doping will certainly get the full support of the UCI,' McQuaid said. 'There is real change going on and some people are resisting it, but I am convinced that the good will win out.'

I walked up the steps from the Tube station into the sunlit canyon of Victoria Street, paused my iPod and slid my sunglasses onto the top of my head. For a while, I just stood and stared.

Thousands of people – Ken Livingstone's multicultural sea of Londoners – clutching Tour de France memorabilia, filled the wide road stretching ahead of me. Britain had embraced the Tour. It was going to be a success after all. The churlish begrudging editorials, on both sides of the English Channel, had been proven wrong.

I battled through the crowds in Parliament Square, crammed five deep against the barriers, waiting expectantly for the first riders to leave the start ramp. I bumped into the normally implacable Steve Taylor of Transport for London, his face flushed from the hot sunshine, eyes wide with excitement, jabbering about the size of the crowds. But he had good reason – the West End streets were jammed with people who had come to see the Tour de France.

It was overwhelming. A tunnel of humanity hemmed in the riders as they sped along the prologue route, through Hyde Park and St James's and back into the Mall. The storybook ending, a Wiggins prologue win, with Millar hot on his heels, didn't materialise. Instead, it was Fabien Cancellara who took the first yellow jersey of 2007. But it didn't matter one bit. After the race, a beaming Christian Prudhomme, director of the Tour, appeared on British TV, and struggled to find the right words to capture the moment.

'Eet was sooo . . . *naice*,' he finally came up with, as if steeped in the sayings of Borat.

Millar, off the pace in the prologue, was missing something. He found it the next morning, in the first road stage, when he left the peloton behind and rode out into Kent at the head of the Tour, cheers ringing in his ears.

We drove across country and joined the race near Tunbridge Wells, rolling slowly through the shady lanes, listening to the updates on Millar's breakaway on Radio Tour. Beneath our wheels, MILLAR was regularly chalked on the road. We stopped to talk to one group of fans. 'He's out the front, is he? Bloody brilliant!' one said. Didn't they care that he'd doped? 'Course not – he's the most honest one out there,' we were told.

Further up the road, a group of giggling children had white-washed bicycles and flags on the tarmac, while in a show of unbridled patriotism, another MILLAR appeared, this time alongside HAMILTON and HENMAN. The smell of British barbecues wafted through the warm afternoon air.

On the few short climbs, heading through the Garden of England and on towards the finish at Canterbury, thousands stood at the roadside, craning their necks to see the race convoy pass. Millar kept up his attack for most of the stage, but faltered before the finish, as the peloton picked up speed and then overhauled him.

All the same, he'd done enough to bag the lead in the King of the Mountains competition, for the first time in his career. Afterwards, he appeared in the team bus compound beyond the stage finish, a faux-smug grin on his face, swaggering around like a teenager in the leading climber's polka-dot jersey.

Disappointed by his prologue result, he had ridden the stage motivated by childhood memories. 'I can remember coming to watch the Tour in 1994, when I was a kid, up against the barriers in Brighton, waiting for four hours. Two riders came through and then ten minutes later, Chris Boardman attacked on his own – it made my whole day.

'I wanted to say thank you to everybody – it was the one opportunity in my life to do that. There were flags everywhere and my name painted on the road,' he said. 'I wanted to stop and say hello to everyone. It was amazing.'

Millar was right. The opening two days of the 2007 Tour were amazing. For a moment, we were innocents again. All there was, the whole weekend, was sunshine.

The fantasy of a clean Tour and, even more fantastically, of a French winner – French national champion Christophe Moreau was enjoying inspired form – persisted until Michael Rasmussen's stage win high in the Alps, among the tower blocks of Tignes.

Ironically, it wasn't Rasmussen who lowered the tone – although he proved well equipped to do that later – but one of the riders presented in Majorca as among Bob Stapleton's generation of 'fresh, clean faces'. The news that Patrik Sinkewitz of T-Mobile had tested positive for testosterone, in an out-of-competition drugs test on 8 June, broke as the race arrived in Tignes.

Like every other rider in the Tour peloton, Sinkewitz had signed a UCI charter renouncing doping and agreeing to forfeit a year's salary in the event of a positive test. This was yet another empty promise.

When news of the positive test broke, Sinkewitz, having finished the stage to Tignes, was riding back down the mountainside to his hotel. The fates hadn't finished with him. He collided with a spectator on the descent and woke up in hospital. That afternoon, the German cycling scene and T-Mobile's battered sponsorship crashed with him.

In Germany, public service broadcasters ARD and ZDF suspended their coverage of the Tour. 'We talked about this with the German teams before the Tour,' Günter Struve, head of programming at ARD, said. 'They assured us that everybody was clean. Our beliefs and confidence have been altered.'

From then on, however good a spin he put on it, Bob Stapleton was struggling. 'He's been caught and that's healthy for the sport,' he said. 'It's good for the sport in the long term. The team is completely devastated because they really believe in the team's policy – they're heartbroken about this.'

ARD, which itself had sponsored T-Mobile in the past, was unimpressed. 'Our contract stated that we would broadcast the Tour as a competition of clean riders, not of people using doping substances,' a spokesman said.

The Sinkewitz Affair was merely an aperitif, however. Michael Rasmussen, with his nervous darting eyes and his evasive manner, was about to take centre stage.

Before the 2007 Tour, the UCI's new anti-doping czar, Anne Gripper, had spoken of a group of riders who trained in plain clothing, rather than in their sponsor's outfits, to preserve their anonymity. Gripper's 'Men In Black' were shady characters, apparently hoping to avoid recognition when based in the locale of their personal 'sports doctors'. One of their tactics was rumoured to be logging false whereabouts details in an effort to avoid out-of-competition testing.

The Danish media had doubts about Rasmussen. It emerged that he had been dropped by his national federation, the Danish Cycling Union (DCU), for missing out-of-competition tests. In the days after he had taken the race lead in Tignes, the pressure on him grew. Later in the week, as the Tour convoy rolled out of Montpellier, the Dane was reduced to banging on the window of race director Christian Prudhomme's car, saying: 'I've done nothing wrong . . .'

Perhaps if he had been placed ninth overall, with no hope of final victory, Rasmussen might have been left alone. But it was less than a year after Operación Puerto and the Landis case remained unfinished business. Nobody wanted Rasmussen in the yellow jersey, leading the Tour through the mountains, seemingly poised for victory.

He was not popular in the peloton either. He rarely shared a room with a teammate and often argued with team mechanics over their refusal to adopt weight-reducing tricks on his equipment. One row was said to have been over a thin layer of paint applied to the handlebars of his bike. Lars Werge saw him as an isolated obsessive, estranged even from some of his Rabobank teammates. The skeletal climber, he recalled, 'counted every grain of rice', and even poured water, rather than milk, on his muesli. 'He's very intense,' Lars said.

The Danish tabloids kept up the pursuit. They claimed that Rasmussen had missed up to four out-of-competition tests, under the jurisdiction of both the DCU and the UCI. His sponsor, Rabobank, mounted a half-hearted defence, but even they sounded like they didn't want him in the race any more. Rasmussen protested his innocence, telling journalists time and time again that he would only answer questions about racing. Catcalls and booing characterised both his appearances on the finish-line podium and in post-race press conferences. Typically, his peers sat on the fence, but David Millar articulated the thoughts of many riders about Rasmussen's continued presence.

'He started the race knowing what would happen but did nothing to rectify the situation. Now we are all screwed, and the Tour is in the shit,' Millar said. 'He took no notice of warnings from the UCI. He has either been unprofessional or has used the system.'

His 'You can trust me' comment haunted Rasmussen. Further allegations against him surfaced, although again he refuted them. Whitney Richards, who had raced mountain bikes alongside him, claimed that in 2002 the Dane had asked him to take a box, containing cycling shoes, to Italy with him. When Richards chose to dump the box in order to pack the shoes away, he claimed to have found bags of an American-branded blood substitute.

Richards said that, after consulting with a physiologist friend, he poured the blood bags away. 'There was no way that I would carry that onto an airplane or through customs for anyone.'

Still, Rasmussen didn't want to talk about it. 'I will only answer questions about the race,' he said.

Richards waved away suggestions that he was merely jealous of the Dane's success. 'It's not that. It was the press conference that got to me. Someone asked him about Bjarne Riis' involvement with drugs and he went on about how he's clean and then added, "You can trust me." That's what set me off.'

Everybody knew that Rasmussen should never have started the Tour. Now, with only the Pyrenees remaining, the prospect of him winning in Paris was becoming all too real. The UCI wrung their hands, as ASO railed against them, and both struggled to justify their inaction over his missed tests.

'In late June, we wrote to Rasmussen and told him that he was on his last chance,' McQuaid said. 'His team Rabobank received a letter reiterating those concerns. But no rules have been broken. All we could do was ask the team to exclude him.

The guy has a right to race and his team has a right to put him in the race. If Rasmussen wins, there will be question marks over the credibility of his victory, but we cannot operate on the basis of media rumours,' McQuaid said.

Erik Breukink, a senior team manager with Rabobank, denied that the team had ever received any communications from the UCI. 'We never heard anything from anybody at the UCI,' Breukink said. 'If they wanted to, they should have suspended him. They shouldn't put responsibility on the teams. ASO points the finger at the UCI and the UCI points back at us.'

Stalemate smothered the race. But there was always another suspect waiting in the wings. Alexander Vinokourov of Kazakhstan, riding for the Astana team and client of Michele Ferrari, was another of the UCI's 'Men in Black'.

Vinokourov had expected to win the Tour, but a crash in the first week left him with knees cut so deeply that he could barely walk. He struggled on but lost time, finally breaking down on the finish line in Briançon. Yet 'Vino' was about to make an 'heroic' comeback. He unleashed an incredible display of power to win the fifty-four kilometre individual time trial, based on a circuit around Albi. If it hadn't been for Cadel Evans of Australia taking second place, Vinokourov's Astana team would have filled the top three placings, with teammates Andrey Kasechkin and Andreas Kloden taking third and fourth. *L'Equipe* hailed his success. '*Le Courage de Vino*', it called it. No wonder one commentator described the paper as 'the *Pravda* of sports journalism'.

And '*Courage*' quickly turned to '*Dopage*' when the news broke in Pau that Vinokourov had tested positive for a blood transfusion.

FULL CIRCLE

'For when the one great scorer comes to write against
your name, he marks – not that you won or lost – but
how you played the game.'

Grantland Rice

The Palais des Congrès in Pau is one of the Tour's more elegant
press rooms. It has grandeur. It also has air conditioning, potted
palms, a coffee bar and restaurant and a panoramic view of the
Pyrenees. There is lots of space for camera crews and photographers. It's a good place for a stand-off, as Lance Armstrong
and David Walsh found out.

Seven years after that confrontation, Michael Rasmussen
steeled himself to face a similar inquisition. If the Dane had
hoped to clarify his situation over his attitude to testing procedures
and to emulate Armstrong's firm rebuttal of doping allegations, he
had been poorly advised. The Chicken turned out to be no match
for Big Tex.

The curtains had been drawn behind Rasmussen to cut out
the bright sunlight behind him, the lights dimmed in the Palais
des Congrès. It gave his doomed press conference a funereal air.
His team's lawyer, Harro Knijff, sat on one side, his Rabobank
manager, Theo de Rooij, on the other.

Rasmussen maintained that he had only failed to comply with
anti-doping regulations through what he described as administrative errors. 'I have made a mistake,' he said. 'The UCI has
given me a recorded warning for the administrative mistake that
I have made. I accept that and I take full responsibility for it. I

am sorry that this situation is coming out now, when I am wearing the yellow jersey. It's harming a sport that I dearly love and it's harming the Tour de France.

'I want to make it absolutely clear that I have had out-of-competition tests prior to the Tour de France and up until this morning I have had fourteen anti-doping tests during the Tour,' Rasmussen said. 'All the results are negative. I support my team and my sponsor Rabobank in the fight against doping and for a clean sport.'

Then the questions started. Very quickly, Rasmussen lost us. The jumble of excuses and justifications only made things worse. Yes, he had received letters warning him over his conduct, yes, he had held a racing licence in Mexico and Monaco – and, in two and a half years, had never undergone any doping controls in either country – and yes, he had mixed up names and dates and refused to accept the jurisdiction of his own anti-doping agency in Denmark.

So what about his written warning from the UCI in March 2006 over his failure to comply with the whereabouts programme? Rasmussen stated that he had telephoned Anne Gripper, UCI anti-doping services manager, on 2 April to apologise. It sounded plausible – except that Anne Gripper only started working for the UCI on 17 October of that year.

One of the Danish journalists immediately called Gripper to ask if she had spoken to Rasmussen in April 2006. 'That would be very difficult,' she replied. 'I stopped working in Australia in January that year and was on holiday until October, when I started working for the UCI.'

When he stood up to leave, Rasmussen looked as drained, as emptied as he would have done after riding the toughest mountain stage of his life. As he walked out through the door, the curtains were pulled open and the sun flooded in.

An hour or so later, David Millar, team manager Mauro Gianetti and assorted Saunier Duval staff appeared in the Palais. The team was to hold a press conference to publicise their efforts to support a reforestation scheme in Mali. Talk of conservation was soon forgotten, though. News of Alexander Vinokourov's positive test whipped through the air, and a sudden frenzy of activity was punctuated by beeping, trilling phones.

Then Daniel Friebe told David the news about Vinokourov. Millar looked overwhelmed. 'We may as well pack our bags and go home,' he said.

The press conference ended in disarray. David got wearily to his feet. His teammates, Iban Mayo and Christophe Rinero, largely ignored, strolled out into the late afternoon sunshine. Gianetti moved towards Millar and said something into his ear. Before he'd finished, a huddle of journalists, largely English-speaking, had formed around them.

Millar looked defeated, not by the questions, which – like every question he'd faced for almost three years – were about doping, but by this latest little death. Kimmage moved in, stern-faced but triumphant, Millar, now staked out before him, beaten. *What would he say now to defend the sport, to defend himself? What could he say?* The moments between them were an empty victory for Kimmage. Millar, his bête noire, seemed finally and irretrievably broken.

I watched. *But there must be more, surely – there must be one more way to turn the screw . . .*

Justin Davis from AFP tossed in a question about doping in other sports. Before Millar could answer, Kimmage, unable to help himself, turned on Davis. 'Let's sort this sport out first,' he snapped.

I didn't blame Millar – not any more. Blaming David again and again, was like blaming a factory chicken for getting fat. A gap had opened between Kimmage and I again, despite the persuasiveness of his evangelical zeal. There was no vindication to be found in this mess. Millar had cheated but he had a conscience; he had not doped without anguish, unlike so many others – even his worst enemies acknowledged that. Even Philippe Gaumont had seen that.

The huddle split up. Kimmage strode off. Millar swooned and looked unsteady, composure lost, his eyes darting around the room. I went up to him. 'Are you alright?' I said.

He stared at me and then, eyes filling, sat down: 'I just feel like crying.'

After that, I didn't see Kimmage's David Millar, the duplicitous doper, the defender of the cheats, the liar and the traitor. I just saw my old friend – the kid pressed against the barriers in Brighton, waiting for Chris Boardman – exhausted, wrung out, drained, ageing in front of me, weeping in a corner of the press room. And so, I put my arm around his shoulders and did my best to console him.

Kimmage hadn't finished with him, though. He crucified Millar's show of emotion in the next weekend's *Sunday Times* – 'tears for a cheat', he called them. I wasn't alone in being amazed by what he wrote.

The next day, Michael Rasmussen's last in the 2007 Tour, the Danish climber won the mountain stage to the summit of the Col d'Aubisque in the Pyrenees. I sat alongside Lars Werge on a grassy bank, a few paces away from the press tent, and watched Rasmussen, Alberto Contador, Levi Leipheimer and Cadel Evans climb through a steep hairpin below us.

Higher up the mountain, the police were waiting on the finish line, not for Rasmussen, but for Bradley Wiggins' teammate, Cristian Moreni. The Cofidis rider, fifty-fourth overall in the Tour, had tested positive for testosterone after the stage to Montpellier. That night, the police turned their attention to the rest of the Cofidis team, searching team vehicles, personal belongings and hotel rooms in Pau.

Eric Boyer, general manager of Cofidis, withdrew the squad from the race. The decision left Wiggins, just three days from completing his first Tour, in a rage. I rang his mobile. No response. Then I noticed that Millar and his team were in the same hotel, so I called him.

'The *flics* are still here, taking the place apart. It's horrible,' he said. Must be bringing back some great memories, I replied. 'Yeah,' said David, before adding with black humour, 'I think I recognise one or two of them . . .'

As Wiggins and his teammates cursed Moreni, Rasmussen was also being told to pack his bags. He had become entangled in his own web. Italian TV commentator, Davide Cassani, said that he had encountered Rasmussen training in the Dolomites in June, even though the Dane had told his team and the UCI that he was out of reach, training in Mexico.

Exasperated, Theo de Rooij confronted his team leader. Then he sacked him. Rasmussen disappeared into the night. 'He lied to me, that is the chief reason for sacking him,' de Rooij said. As he exited under cover of darkness, Rasmussen described his team boss as 'mad'.

'He is at the end of his tether,' Rasmussen said. 'I wasn't in Italy, no way. That's the story of one man who thinks he saw me. But there's not the slightest proof.'

There was little joy in his downfall on the part of the Danish journalists, who had pursued Rasmussen so relentlessly. 'I have had some hate mail and threats,' Lars told me, wearily. 'But by the end, Rasmussen seemed to think he could walk on water.'

'Taking drugs makes your life worse. It changes you. It turns you into an animal or a monster. It changes your face, it changes your attitude. It takes over your soul. You turn into a con artist who has to lie every day. Only some guys can deal with it. Guys like me and Pantani can't. I have been much luckier than Pantani, because I was able to save myself and he never could.'

Matt DeCanio, American cyclist and whistle-blower

There was never a golden age of fair play in cycling's history. Cheating has always been a characteristic of the sport and particularly of the Tour de France. A hundred years ago, riders used to hop on trains to make up for their shortcomings. These days, they scour the Internet for suppliers and information on new products.

There was not any single moment when I finally realised that a sport – an obsession – that had helped me come to terms with my own dark places and to rebuild my life, had in fact become a prison of its own. Instead, my faith in those working within cycling died slowly – the 'death of a thousand cuts' – as scandal followed scandal, until there was no residue of faith left.

The values that had once reeled me in became distorted in a tight-knit world where decency, where doing the right thing, was regarded as naive, eccentric and futile. In this brutalised environment you had to make a choice; speak out and risk alienation, or keep your mouth shut and stay in the club. The repeated failures to change that cultural malaise were exhausting.

For me, those who have doped, endorsed doping or failed to condemn it have made a business choice, not an ethical one. The spread of that culture reflects a collective failure of responsibility that has diminished the Tour de France in every way. It has made the race a bad – even a deadly – joke.

In a problematic world, sport should offer escape; it should offer sanctuary from the casual lies and banal cruelties that punctuate everyday life. Rather than embodying the ugliest elements in human nature, it should strive to encapsulate the best.

We love sport, not for its certainties, but for its uncertainties. But uncertainty is of no use to a doper. They want guarantees of success. They hate the unknown: consistency, day in day out, year in year out, is everything for them, because they are desperate to maintain their position.

There are many team bosses, riders, coaches and promoters, who discovered their consciences only when it became financially expedient to do so. Others lost their moral compass long ago, so brutalised did they become by everyday cheating. Those people will never welcome change.

Dopers cheat us, and falsify our memories – they take the sport out of our sport. Their use of doping renders our experience meaningless. It seems that there is no moral imperative that can be brought to bear to dissuade them. Appealing to the athlete's conscience has proven to be laughably naive, particularly in cycling where doping was ubiquitous.

'It was like white noise,' David Millar said of the world he inhabited. 'The question was not "Why did I dope?" but "Why didn't I dope sooner?"'

Paradoxically, dopers are fragile, paranoid and insecure, because they know that, on the day they don't dope, they will have no certainty. Their status hangs by a thread, reliant on their supplier, their doctor, their network. Ironically, for people who have given their lives to the pursuit of sporting excellence, those who dope themselves will never really know what their natural limits are, both as an athlete and a human being. Doping is a tragic experience for them: it takes away the experience of their true identity, of their true capabilities.

The elements that came together in the mid 1990s – ineffective doping controls, an increasingly punishing racing calendar, a heightened level of media interest, a new business ethic allied to unprecedented levels of corporate investment, a global village of television and internet followers and an ineffectual governing body – led cycling into the abyss in which it has found itself.

In this climate, sport fans veer between denial and anger, posting endless rants on message boards and in blogs, their desire for truth pulled this way and that. Their patience has been tested to breaking point, their investment betrayed, their loyalty gone unrewarded. Yet so strong is their love of the sport, and in particular of the Tour, that they still want to believe. They deserve better.

Ultimately, what happens next is our responsibility.

Will we still retain our passion for professional sport if we believe that most of the performances are chemically enhanced? Will television companies still want to pay millions of dollars for the rights to legendary events, such as the Tour de France, or the Olympic Games, if audiences have become disenchanted? Will global corporations want to invest in sport if what sets it apart – its credibility as *sport* – collapses?

Who cares, *who cares*, if what we see is a show? Why does doping really matter? Why not level the playing field and legalise all products? Isn't doping simply the inevitable consequence of a drug-dependent, technologically enhanced modern society, that embraces plastic surgery, is Ecstasy-tolerant, Viagra-fuelled – in short, aren't all of us *doped* in some way or another?

Yes – a lot of us are, but the perversion of drug use in sport is that these athletes are not sick or injured, but are using products to go beyond their genetic limits, to achieve fraudulent success. There are other practical issues – the health of athletes, the health of the public, fraud and legality, addiction, trafficking – and there is the most basic morality: doping is cheating.

Legalisation of doping in sport would, as Dick Pound said, be 'an abandonment of all ethical and moral responsibility'.

'It's a downward spiral,' Pound believes. 'If you legalise things at the top, then it becomes legal all the way down through the system. You're going to get fourteen- and fifteen-year-olds using EPO and HGH in industrial quantities. And if that happened, and if I were a parent with a child thinking of playing competitive sport, I'd say, "Let's do something else – it's not worth what you'd have to do to yourself."'

We no longer expect athletes to refrain from doping because of a crisis of conscience, because it is cheating, because it is fraudulent, because ultimately it is wrong. We expect them to refrain because they may get caught, sanctioned, fined, humiliated, banned.

In the end that is the greatest loss of innocence: that we now expect them to at least try to dope. So because we cannot trust them, we have to police them, to monitor their movements. We DNA test them; we take hair, blood and urine samples to store for the future; we rouse them at dawn for yet more testing. We don't believe in them, or in their word, any more.

The testing is to help us believe; to prove that all is well, that they are clean – not that they are doped, because we assume that without those safeguards in place they automatically would be. The testing is in place to maintain the illusion of fair play.

And after all that, when they have been cleared to compete and they emerge from the secretive cocoons of their hotel rooms, air-conditioned buses and private jets and finally start competing, it's a reasonable question to ask yourself: *what happened to the sport?*

The 2007 Tour de France made it to Paris, just.

Spanish rider Alberto Contador, clad in the yellow jersey, smiled and waved on the Champs-Elysées podium, even as most of France turned its back in disdain. Johan Bruyneel had led a team to Tour victory for the eighth year. There was a certain symmetry that a team forced to sack its leader, Ivan Basso, because of doping, should then win the Tour because a rival team, Rabobank, was also forced to sack its leader, Michael Rasmussen, for missing random drug tests. It was a convoluted, dysfunctional story, typical of the modern Tour. And as Contador and Bruyneel celebrated, the suppressed whispers of doping that had characterised the era had become white noise.

By the end of the following month, even after eight Tour wins, through Armstrong and Contador, Tailwind Sports, the Discovery Channel team's management company, had quit the sport and renounced the search for new sponsors. 'We were in talks with a number of companies about the opportunity and were confident a new sponsor was imminent,' Bill Stapleton said. 'We have chosen, however, to end those discussions.'

In the aftermath of that decision, Lance Armstrong distanced himself from the sport. 'Clearly things need to improve on many levels, with a more unified front, before you would see us venture back into cycling,' he said. By the end of September 2007, the Texan went further, telling the media that a continuing interest in cycling was 'just a distraction for me'.

Bruyneel announced his retirement. 'I've achieved everything that I could in the sport,' he said. 'I've always said that I wanted to stop on top and I think it's the right time.' But then the Astana team came calling and the Belgian reversed his retirement plans, becoming a Kazakh Bob Stapleton, charged with leading the ethical makeover that would make Astana palatable once again to the Tour organisation.

But the makeover didn't take. Seven months later, after Bruyneel had taken over the Astana team that had quit the 2007 Tour in disgrace after Alexander Vinokourov's positive test, the Tour de France organisation banned Astana from its events.

Not even his status as defending Tour champion could earn Alberto Contador and Astana a reprieve. His co-leader, Levi Leipheimer, set up a campaign to overturn his exile called 'Let

Levi Ride'. The decision to ban Astana was draconian, but, given their past transgressions, wholly deserved. Nonetheless, it split the sport once more.

Only cycling has been so bitterly divided by the war on drugs. Athletics, in the wake of the BALCO Affair and the downfall of Marion Jones, appears increasingly polarised, yet in most other sports, journalists can still cosy up to the top stars without questioning their ethics on a daily basis. As the crisis deepened in cycling, that became impossible. Doping forced us all to choose where we stood.

Looking back, it took a very long time for me to become faithless. The ubersceptics no doubt rolled their eyes in despair at my resistance to finally giving up the ghost. Yet eventually, the sport's inability to achieve change angered me. At the same time, I realised how polluted my own life had been by the melancholy and defeatism of doping. Acknowledging the extent of that contamination was a liberation of sorts.

The essence of doping is cheating and the essence of cheating is defeatism. Doping says, 'This can't be done any other way; this can't be achieved through hard work or talent, through intelligence, determination and honesty.' All that's left is to lie and cheat and to make others complicit to that cheating.

And living and working in an environment where those values are the currency of everyday relationships, kills you a little. It colours your belief and taints your faith in human nature. That's how the contagion of cheating works, how the acceptance of it as a value system spreads.

It doesn't matter that it was cycling: it could have been athletics, rugby, cricket, football, politics or corporate business. Much of life is tainted by corruption at some levels. My journey from adoring fan to embittered insider, was beautiful and bewildering, privileged and, finally, poisonous.

'Are you bitter?' Paul Kimmage texted me, after we had met in London that day.

I thought about it for a while. 'Yes – who wouldn't be?' I replied.

Cycling still exerts a fascination for me. Every now and then I pull on some Lycra and head out into the Sussex Downs to tackle Ditchling Beacon, the toughest climb on the opening days of the 1994 Tour and a hill that every English cyclist knows well. The paint is fading now, but the last time I weaved my way up to the top, you could still make out PANTANI stencilled onto the road, just before you struggle over the windswept ridge to be greeted by a view of Brighton and the grey sea.

I didn't ask to see the syringes at my feet, to hear the tearful confessions, to endure the tedious denials of Virenque, Hamilton, Landis, Basso, Riis and the rest. I didn't go looking for the confrontations, the isolations, the disputes. But they became the currency of my everyday existence, an inescapable part of life on Tour. That experience changed me. I realised that I could never go back to the way we were – Bernard, Greg and I – in the twilight hours of a rented room, ignorant and enraptured, out on the wild and beautiful Croix de Fer, our dreams fused together on the tattered tape of a VCR.

EPILOGUE

In July 2006, twelve months after retiring from racing, with the Discovery Channel team appearing lost and directionless without him, Lance Armstrong came back to the Tour de France. He made a flying visit to the Alps, hanging out with his ex-teammates and touring the late-night bars with Jake Gyllenhaal and their entourage.

A few days before leaving for Europe, Armstrong had joked on American TV that the French football team had tested positive – 'for being assholes'. This came within hours of the nation's 2006 World Cup Final defeat and the career-ending dismissal of Zinedine Zidane.

When Lance's private jet touched down at the foot of the Alps, the locals gave him a warm reception. 'It was a joke – where's your sense of humour?' he retorted when challenged by French television. But a reservoir of resentment spilled over. Tabloid newspaper *France-Soir* paid the seven-time Tour champion back in spades.

'*Bienvenue en France, Trou-duc!*' it bellowed. 'Welcome to France, Asshole!'

When he got to Alpe d'Huez, he held court with a group of favoured journalists. One of them asked him if he had been offended by the *France-Soir* headline.

Lance Armstrong looked around the room, at the familiar faces, at the notebooks, cameras and tape recorders, poised, ready and waiting, and threw his head back and laughed.

ACKNOWLEDGEMENTS

This book was originally entitled *Ten Years in a Hire Car*, which, I have to say, I still rather like. However, with doping now the dominant issue in cycling (and other sports), such a jolly title became increasingly inappropriate. *Bad Blood* was far more fitting.

For their guidance and support I owe thanks to my agent, David Luxton, to Tristan Jones and all at Random House. I'd also particularly like to thank Daniel Friebe for being such a good friend and collaborator over the past few years, during late nights on the road and a few lost days on the golf course.

For inspiration, support and provocation, thanks to the following: my family, Murf and Ted, Aubrey and Joan, Fergus MacLeod, Steven Hunter, Freya North, Alun Williams and Sally O'Sullivan, Andy Hood, Rupert Guinness, Justin Davis, Sam Abt, Bob Chicken Snr, Ellis Bacon, Lars Werge, William Fotheringham, Rowan Andrews, Alastair Campbell, Hedwig Kroener, Susanne Horsdal, Phil O'Connor, Bonnie de Simone, Graham Jones and Simon Brotherton, Mick Bennett, Ian Banbery, Sarah Wynne, David Chappell, Stephen Penman, Richard Moore, Tim Moore, Deirdre Rooney and Sarah Wharton, Andrew and Judith Hodge, Chris Boardman, Rufus, Leslie, Neil and Josh, Avril, Frances and David Millar, James and Lindsay Poole, Peter Cossins, Les Woodland, David Poole, James Warren, Pete Goding and Paul Godfrey, Lance Armstrong, Brendan Gallagher, Kenny Pryde, Duncan Steer, Paul Auster, Matt Rendell, Kirsten Begg, Julian Clark, David Sharp, Ruth Jarvis, Paul Kimmage, Pierre Ballester, Denis Descamps, Greg LeMond, Wes Anderson, Tim Lott and Jonathan Coe, Matt DeCanio, Chris Lillywhite, Frankie Andreu and Filippo Simeoni, all those at the roadside, the hoteliers and barmen and so many others, who really are far too numerous to mention.